HORMONE REPLACEMENT THERAPY AND THE ENDOMETRIUM

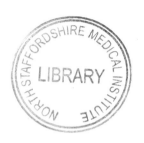

HORMONE REPLACEMENT THERAPY AND THE ENDOMETRIUM

Edited by

Farook Al-Azzawi, MA, PhD, FRCOG
and May Wahab, MD, MRCOG

Gynaecology Research Unit, Department of Obstetrics and Gynaecology
University of Leicester, Leicester, UK

The Parthenon Publishing Group
International Publishers in Medicine, Science & Technology

NEW YORK   LONDON

Library of Congress Cataloging-in-Publication Data

Data available on request

Published in the USA by
The Parthenon Publishing Group Inc.
One Blue Hill Plaza
PO Box 1564, Pearl River
New York 10965, USA

Published in the UK and Europe by
The Parthenon Publishing Group Limited
Casterton Hall, Carnforth
Lancs. LA6 2LA, UK

Copyright ©2001 The Parthenon Publishing Group

British Library Cataloguing in Publication Data

Hormone replacement therapy and the endometrium
   1.Endometrium - Diseases - Hormone therapy
   I.al-Azzawi, Farook II.Wahab, May
   618.1′4

ISBN 1850700923

Typeset by Speedlith Group, Manchester, UK
Printed and bound by T. G. Hostench S.A., Spain

Contents

List of Contributors

F. Al-Azzawi, MB ChB, MA (Cantab), PhD, FRCOG
Director, Gynaecology Research Unit
Department of Obstetrics and Gynaecology
University of Leicester
Leicester, UK

M. Habiba, MB ChB, MSc, PhD, MRCOG
Senior Lecturer Consultant
Department of Obstetrics and Gynaecology
University of Leicester
Leicester, UK

A. H. Taylor, MSc, PhD, MRCOG
Molecular Endocrinologist, Gynaecology Research Unit
Department of Obstetrics and Gynaecology
University of Leicester
Leicester, UK

J. R. Thompson, PhD
Professor
Department of Epidemiology
University of Leicester
Leicester, UK

M. Wahab, MB ChB, MD, MRCOG
Specialist Registrar, Gynaecology Research Unit
Department of Obstetrics and Gynaecology
University of Leicester
Leicester, UK

Foreword

The effects of hormone replacement therapy (HRT) on the endometrium are a frequent cause of problems for both the clinician and patient. Ever since the mid-1970s, when a series of reports from North America identified a considerably increased risk of endometrial cancer in women taking unopposed estrogen, the need for additional progestogen in HRT regimens for endometrial protection has been accepted. Sequential regimens of estrogen and progestogen will almost inevitably provoke bleeding, and even if this is regular, predictable and controlled, this is often the cause of patient dissatisfaction. When the bleeding is irregular or too heavy, there is further concern about endometrial disease, but there is widespread uncertainty about how to manage bleeding problems. Unfortunately even a regular and predictable bleed following a conventional dose of progestogen does not give complete reassurance about the state of the endometrium.

Farook Al-Azzawi and his colleagues in Leicester have been investigating the effects of sex steroids on the endometrium and the bleeding patterns generated in postmenopausal women for many years. This book represents a culmination of much of their work, and is produced in a format to provide information for both the scientist and general clinician. It is intriguing that the postmenopausal endometrium seems to respond differently from that which occurs during the premenopausal menstrual cycle, and with advances in molecular medicine and the development of new hormone combinations for HRT, the differential effects on the endometrium are beginning to be explained. There has been some complacency in recent years about the safety of current regimens of HRT, and with an increasing emphasis on longer-term treatment in order to realize significant effects on osteoporosis prevention and possibly cardiovascular disease, it is especially important to be reassured of long-term endometrial safety.

This book provides clear details on how to manage and investigate patients with bleeding problems on HRT, as well as the latest scientific information. It will be of great value and stimulus to all who have an interest in the effect of sex steroids, whether they are working in the laboratory or in the clinic.

David Sturdee, MD, FRCOG
Solihull Hospital, Solihull, UK

Introduction

Today physicians and gynecologists are expected to provide advice and management plans for postmenopausal women to cure symptoms of estrogen deficiency and to prevent subsequent degenerative disorders known to be modulated by a lack of estrogen. This area is covered in Chapter 1. A program of promotion of health and maintenance of quality of life is relatively easily achievable by estrogen-based regimens. These regimens stimulate endometrial growth in the majority of women and result in endometrial bleeding. Given the age of the population in question and the fact that the incidence of neoplastic conditions in post-reproductive years is a function of age, as it peaks a decade after the menopause, the major concern thus far has been the exclusion of neoplasia of the endometrium. Since the majority of women who present with abnormal bleeding do not have cancer, the declaration of a benign endometrium *per se* does not offer these women relief from their symptoms. The postmenopausal population is increasing as a percentage of the population, with higher expectations for healthy aging. The risk:benefit ratio in favor of continuing hormone replacement therapy (HRT) has been consistently documented, and therefore it is expected that the demand for this treatment will increase as well. Consequently, there is a need to explore effective methods to deal with exogenous sex steroid-related menstrual irregularities, so that continuation rates with HRT programs are enhanced.

The aim of this manual is to provide an extract of the experience of the authors in dealing with the endometrium at both clinical and research levels. Methods of assessment of uterine bleeding are largely subjective and variable, and there is little consensus as to how to evaluate menstrual diaries in the clinical setting as well as in drug development studies. The articles in the literature on endometrial bleeding can seldom be compared, since the definitions employed, the size of the samples studied and the length of observation are not uniform. The chapter on statistical evaluation of menstrual events explores methods of assessment of within-woman and between-women variability, which to a large extent explain the apparent discrepancy between the clinical observations and the reported efficacy of hormonal regimens. It also provides statistical explanations and guidance on which factors to consider in forming a research plan in this field.

The histology of the normal endometrium during the natural cycle has been established, but evaluation of the relative impact of individual HRT regimens on individual histologic parameters has not. The chapter on endometrial histology under the influence of sex steroids advocates the construction of a mathematical model to help draw comparisons between the normal endometrium of the natural cycle and those endometria under the influence of different HRT regimens, or the endometrium from women with dysfunctional bleeding.

The advent of molecular medicine is enabling physicians in most specialties to understand many subtleties of pathogenesis and the variable modes of action of an increasing number of therapeutic agents. The ubiquitous nature of the estrogen, and other sex steroid, receptors engages the gynecologist in the whole field of human biology. A review of the current understanding of sex steroid receptors and their interaction and control is incorporated in this book. The chapter on progestogens aims to explore the biochemical relationships between various progestogens available in clinical practice and throw light on the pharmacologic assessment of their potency, thus giving the reader the scientific background to help him or her to deal with these agents.

The clinical aspects of the endometrium in the post-reproductive years are examined in three consecutive chapters. The pathophysiology of dysfunctional bleeding and the potential risk factors for endometrial neoplasia in association with exogenous sex steroids and tamoxifen are discussed in Chapter 7. Investigation of the endometrium is an area riddled with apparently conflicting approaches, and Chapter 8 attempts to address many of these controversies, with an assessment of what is regarded at present as the 'gold standard' of care in this field. The final chapter discusses approaches to the diagnosis and treatment of the menopause, and addresses some of the controversies surrounding the use of HRT in women with cancer of the breast and of the endometrium and in those with a history of venous thromboembolism.

1
Consequences of estrogen deficiency
F. Al-Azzawi

INTRODUCTION

The menopause, the final menstrual period, marks the end of a continuum of declining physiologic fertility. Decreased fertility in relative or absolute terms antedates the menopause by 10–15 years. The climacteric is the period of time (about 4–5 years) around the menopause during which ovarian function is gradually compromised. At the turn of the 20th century life expectancy in women of the Western world was about 58 years; at present it is about 82, but as the mean age of the menopause, 51 years, has not changed, more than one-third of a Western woman's life is expected to occur after the menopause. This is the first time in human history when long postmenopausal existence has been witnessed on such a scale. More importantly, the disability-free life expectancy for the whole population between the ages of 50 and 60 has not changed over the last 30 years[1], the main problems being cardiovascular disease and arthritis. For both genders, aging is the primary factor influencing disabilities related to cardiovascular disease, arthritis, Alzheimer's disease and visual and hearing problems. It is expected that more women disabled by these conditions will survive after the menopause, and that the menopause will be increasingly found to be a confounding variable, the treatment of which may profoundly influence the clinical progress of such disabilities. With the expected increase in the postmenopausal population over the next 30 years, the health issues modulated by the menopause have moved from a peripheral medical interest into a central health care program that commands a different strategy for the allocation of resources and the delivery of services.

PATHOPHYSIOLOGY OF THE MENOPAUSE

From the age of 35 years onwards there is a progressive increase in the level of follicle-stimulating hormone (FSH), indicating a reduced amount of effective estradiol and inhibin B production[2]. In an elegant study which combined data from other reports, the ovarian content of primordial follicles was shown to sustain a sharp decline at about the age of 37 (Figure 1.1)[3,4]. Should this rapid decline in the number of primordial follicles not occur, menstruation could be expected to continue until the age of 70.

The source of estradiol is the granulosa cell layer, which lines the growing primordial follicles. As the number of gonadotropin-responsive primordial follicles declines, and consequently the number of growing granulosa cells, symptoms and signs of estrogen deficiency start to develop, although the dramatic biochemical and tissue structural changes in women appear soon after the menstrual periods cease completely. Owing to the hypergonadotropic state, steroidogenesis continues

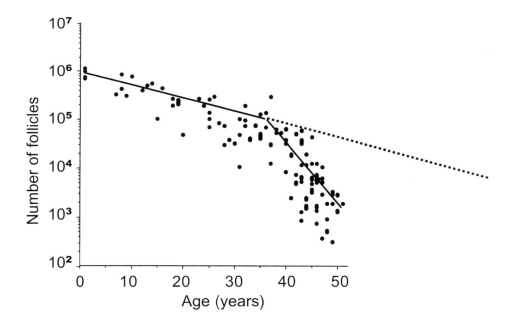

Figure 1.1. Bi-exponential model of declining number of follicles in pairs of human ovaries (age 0–51). ©European Society of Human Reproduction and Embryology. Adapted by permission of Oxford University Press/Human Reproduction, from Faddy MJ, Gosden RG, Gougeon A, *et al. Hum Reprod* 1992;7:1342–6[3]

in the ovarian stroma and theca cells, with an increased production of androgens, particularly androstenedione and testosterone, and to a lesser extent dehydro-epiandrosterone and its sulfate (DHEA and DHEAS), which are peripherally converted into estrone, the predominant (albeit weak) circulating estrogen in the postmenopause.

EFFECTS OF ESTROGEN DEFICIENCY

Table 1.1 shows the symptoms associated with the menopause and postmenopausal years.

Central nervous system

The ubiquitous distribution of the estrogen receptors in many parts of the central nervous system[5] may explain the wide spectrum of symptoms that results from estrogen deprivation. Estrogens regulate the synthesis and the rate of release of many neuropeptides, neurotransmitters, and particularly the noradrenergic trans-mission in the medulla oblongata, and the hypothalamus. Estrogen increases

Table 1.1. Symptoms associated with the climacteric and postmenopausal years

Acute consequences of estrogen deficiency	
Vasomotor symptoms	Hot flushes
	Sweats
	Insomnia
	Palpitations
Psychologic symptoms	Mood changes
	Anxiety
	Loss of memory
	Loss of concentration
	Irritability
Reproductive tract symptoms	Vaginal dryness
	Loss of libido
	Dyspareunia
Urinary symptoms and urethral syndrome	
Chronic consequences of estrogen deficiency	
Skeletal disease: osteoporosis	
Cardiovascular diseases and strokes	

sensory perception, locomotor activity, limb co-ordination and balance[6]. Estrogen deficiency reduces serotonin synthesis in the brain, which may contribute to the development of insomnia[7,8]. In addition estrogen replacement treatment has been associated with a reduction in the incidence of Alzheimer's disease[9,10].

Vasomotor symptoms
One of the immediate effects of estrogen deficiency is the instability of the thermo-regulatory center located in the hypothalamus with the consequent development of hot flushes and sweating (vasomotor symptoms). The hot flush results from sudden vasodilatation of skin capillaries, which typically affects the chest area and spreads upwards to the facial skin; there is an increase in skin temperature by about 1–2°C. This hot flush lasts for less than a minute and is usually followed by perspiration. The majority of women experience vasomotor symptoms of varying degrees of frequency and severity, and as many as 25–50% will continue to suffer from these symptoms 5 years after the menopause. The quality of life may be severely compromised by the presence of menopausal symptoms, which are easily cured by hormone replacement therapy (HRT). It is essential to appreciate that the absence of vasomotor symptoms does not reflect a lesser susceptibility to the degenerative changes elsewhere in the body as a result of the menopause.

Urogenital aging

The loss of estrogen affects the lower genital tract, resulting in thinning of the vaginal epithelium with impaired epithelial maturation (Figure 1.2) and a reduction in vaginal transudates, which causes vaginal dryness and dyspareunia. There is also a reduction in the supporting collagen. A decrease in cervical mucus may further contribute to the symptom of vaginal dryness. The endometrium becomes atrophic. Ligamentous support to the uterus, cervix and vagina undergoes atrophy, which may present clinically as genital prolapse. Atrophy of the urothelium of the trigone of the bladder and of the urethra makes these areas more sensitive to the irritating effect of urine, causing urgency, frequency and dysuria.

Skin

As a result of the aging process as well as hypo-estrogenemia, the skin sustains a reduction in the amount of collagen with thinning of the dermis and consequently promotes the development of wrinkles and the appearance of lines. The use of estrogen increases dermal thickness mainly because of an increase in the thickness of collagen, which retains more water as a result[11,12].

Bone metabolism

Increased osteoclastic activity supervenes within 6–8 weeks of the loss of estrogen, and as a result a number of biochemical changes may be observed:

(1)   Reduction in serum level of osteocalcin;

(2)   Increase in urinary hydroxyproline:creatinine ratio;

(3)   Increase in renal leakage of calcium; and

(4)   Reduction in intestinal absorption of calcium.

Osteoporosis

Osteoporosis is a condition marked by a reduction in bone mass, due to either reduced bone formation or accelerated bone resorption. Bone remodeling is a continuous process of resorption and bone formation, with activated bone resorption being the main feature of estrogen deficiency. The main morphologic change in osteoporosis is the loss of the collagenous framework that constitutes the bone micro-architecture. In the postmenopausal population it is manifested by a progressive reduction in height, development of dorsal kyphosis ('dowager's hump') and by the high incidence of low trauma fractures of the distal radius, vertebral compression and fractures of the neck of the femur.

Fracture risk and osteoporosis

The lifetime risk of osteoporotic fractures for a 50-year-old white man is 2% for vertebral fractures, 2% for distal radius fractures and 3% for femoral neck fractures; the corresponding figures for a woman of the same age and ethnicity are 11, 13 and 14%, respectively[13]. Therefore, more than one-third of women will sustain one or more osteoporotic fracture(s) in their lifetime. The maximum bone mass is attained by the age of 30, followed by a plateau for 5–10 years, after which age-related bone loss of about 0.5% per year ensues[14,15]. At the menopause a phase of accelerated bone loss of about 4% per year has been recognized, which affects mainly cancellous bone and lasts for about 4 years[14,16]. Afterwards the annual rate of bone loss slows back to 1%[17]. By the age of 80 a woman who has not had HRT will have lost 30–50% of her bone mass. A reduction of bone density by one standard deviation, in the hip for example, increases the risk of hip fractures by 2.6-fold[18]. Femoral neck fractures carry a 15% fatality within 3 months and are associated with a high disability rate of survivors. Women of northwestern European extraction and Asian women accrue a lower bone density during their lifetime and are therefore more susceptible to osteoporosis after the menopause, when compared to Afro-Caribbean or Mediterranean women.

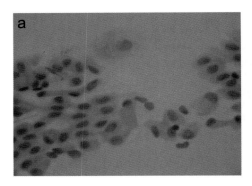 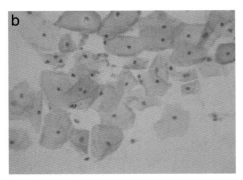

Figure 1.2. Vaginal cytology. (**a**) Vaginal smear obtained from an estrogen-deficient woman showing small rounded parabasal cells with scanty basophilic cytoplasm, which contain large nuclei. (**b**) In premenopausal women, or after estrogen replacement therapy, no less than 20% of the cells obtained at vaginal smear contain large flat eosinophilic squamous epithelial cells with acidophilic cytoplasm and relatively small nuclei

Estrogen effects on bone metabolism

The effects of estrogen on bone metabolism are:

(1) Reduction in interleukin-1 (IL-1) and IL-6 production in bone remodeling units[19];

(2) Induction of apoptosis in osteoclasts[20];

(3) Stimulation of bone formation by the increased production of insulin-like growth factor-I (IGF-I), IGF-II and transforming growth factor-α (TGF-α)[21];

(4) Increased synthesis of calcitonin[22]; and

(5) Increased expression of vitamin D receptors in osteoblasts[23].

Other causes of osteoporosis are listed in Table 1.2.

The cardiovascular system

Estrogen deficiency results in several changes in the cardiovascular system.

Table 1.2. Causes of osteoporosis

Metabolic and endocrine etiology	Hypogonadism
	Hyperadrenocorticism
	Thyrotoxicosis
	Hyperparathyroidism
Nutritional deficiencies	Vitamin D deficiency
	Alcoholism
	Malabsorption syndrome
	Chronic liver disease
Drug-induced	Chronic corticosteroid use
	Chronic heparin therapy

The heart

Ischemic heart disease (IHD) is the most common cause of death in women over the age of 55, and accounts for about 25% of deaths. The menopause is an independent risk factor for IHD, the overall relative risk in the menopause being 2.7, a risk that increases with younger age at menopause[24]. In women with a previous myocardial infarction (MI), ever-use of estrogen significantly reduces the age-adjusted mortality from a repeat MI to 0.56 (95% confidence interval (CI), 0.50–0.61)[25]. The relative risk for cardiovascular disease in women on estrogen replacement remains 0.65 even after adjustment for other risk factors: previous MI, diabetes, hypertension, smoking, cholesterol, body mass index (BMI), age and education[26].

There are structural and functional changes in the heart following the menopause:

(1) Reduced stroke volume[27];

(2) Reduced cardiac output[28];

(3) Left ventricular hypertrophy: posterior wall and septum thickness increases by 10% within 5 years postmenopause[29]; and

(4) Higher incidence of 'ischemia minor' in the electrocardiograms of oophorectomized women[30].

A reduction in the incidence of cardiovascular disease, including cerebrovascular accidents, will therefore have the greatest potential to influence the life expectancy of women. Preventing myocardial ischemia, non-fatal infarctions and cerebrovascular insufficiency ranks among the most important ways of increasing the 'disability-free life expectancy' of women.

Blood pressure

The incidence of hypertension is significantly higher in hypo-estrogenic post-menopausal women when compared to women receiving estrogen replacement therapy after adjustment for age, race and weight[31]. Postmenopausal estrogen replacement treatment reduces systolic and diastolic blood pressure in women, an effect which is not dose-related. In addition estrogen reduces the stress-induced rise in blood pressure. The arterial vasodilatory effect of estrogen may be a crucial mechanism in modulating its cardiovascular protective effects, whether that is due to increased prostacyclin production[32], calcium channel blockade[33] or endothelium-independent vaso-relaxation[34].

The effect of estrogen on blood pressure has been reported in many publications. An elevation in blood pressure, as measured by the conventional sphygmomanometer, was documented by some workers[35], a rise ascribed by some to the type of estrogen used[36]. Others failed to demonstrate a change in blood pressure with estrogen therapy in normotensive or in hypertensive women[37,38]. A reduction in blood pressure was documented in a double-blind crossover study of conjugated equine estrogens and placebo[39]. Automated ambulatory blood pressure measurement is a useful technique to overcome the problem of 'white coat' hypertension, and gives a number of readings throughout a 24-hour period. In a comparative study which evaluated the mean change in daytime and night-time systolic and diastolic blood pressure in oophorectomized women there was a consistent drop in systolic and diastolic blood pressure during the day and night. This trend was statistically significant in women treated with transdermal estradiol compared to oral estrogen after 6 months of observation[40]. Following oral administration of estrogen the induction of angiotensinogen through the first pass effect on the liver has been proposed, but this has not been substantiated in the literature. Certain gene polymorphisms may be responsible for the development of high blood pressure in some estrogen users; however, this has not yet been documented.

Effects of estrogens on blood vessels

Postmenopausal estrogen therapy results in an acceleration of blood flow in the aorta[41], reduced peripheral vascular resistance[42] and a significant increase in the pulsatility index in the carotid arteries[43]. Postmenopausal estrogen supplement delays the onset of exercise-induced ST-depression and improved exercise tolerance in women with angiographically confirmed IHD[44], and angiographic studies have shown a reduced risk of coronary artery occlusion in estrogen users[45].

Cerebrovascular effect of estrogen
A sex difference exists in cerebral blood flow, being greater in the premenopause than in age-matched males, but it declines to equality after the menopause[46]. Estrogen treatment in the postmenopause reduces resistance in the internal carotid artery[43] and middle cerebral artery[47]. In another study the use of unopposed estrogen in women with established carotid artery atheromas resulted in a reduction of 28% of plaque length and 18% of plaque thickness after 6 months' treatment[48].

Lipoprotein metabolism
Lipid metabolism is a complex process which involves mainly the liver, adipose tissue, skeletal muscles and peripheral blood monocytes in addition to the intestinal villi (Figure 1.3). The disturbance in lipid metabolism ranks highly among the identified risk factors of atherosclerosis and cardiovascular disease. Elevated serum levels of total cholesterol and triglycerides have been shown to have a linear positive relationship, and high-density lipoprotein (HDL)-cholesterol has been found to have an inverse relationship with the risk of IHD.

There are sex differences in lipid profile, which in women is profoundly affected by hormonal changes. Prior to the menopause women have a less atherogenic lipid profile, but the changes in lipoprotein metabolism in postmenopausal women have been associated with the increased cardiovascular mortality. The risk has been shown to decline with the lowering of serum cholesterol[49].

After the menopause women retain their higher level of HDL-cholesterol, but this is counteracted by a higher level of low-density lipoprotein (LDL)-cholesterol than in men. About half the patients with coronary artery disease have reduced HDL-cholesterol levels, the commonest lipoprotein abnormality. Consequently elevation of HDL-cholesterol by estrogen treatment should be viewed as an important vehicle for the cardioprotective effect of this hormone. Estrogen reduces LDL-cholesterol oxidation and therefore interferes with its uptake by monocytes and tissue macrophages, a particularly important step in the development of atherosclerosis. The significance of raised serum triglycerides as an independent risk factor for cardiovascular disease is still controversial. About 30–50% of the

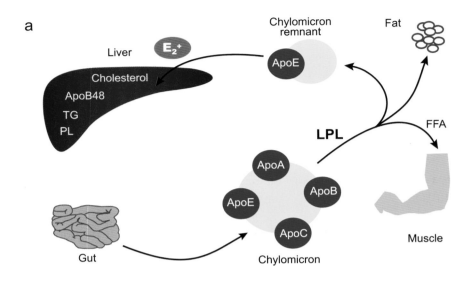

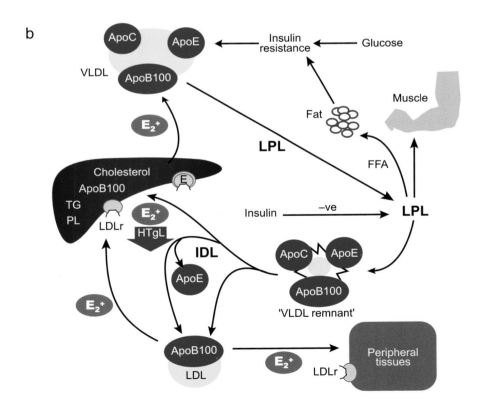

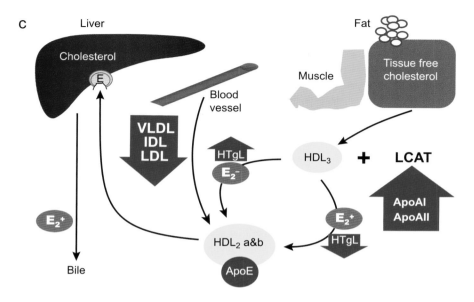

Figure 1.3. Effect of estrogen on lipid metabolism. (**a**) Estrogen and exogenous lipid transport. (**b**) Estrogen and endogenous lipid transport. (**c**) Estrogen and reverse cholesterol transport. Apo, apolipoprotein; E_2, estradiol; FFA, free fatty acids; HDL, high-density lipoprotein; HTgL, hepatic triglyceride lipase; IDL, intermediate-density lipoprotein; LCAT, lecithin–cholesterol acyltransferase; LDL, low-density lipoprotein; LDLr, LDL receptor; LPL, lipoprotein lipase; PL, phospholipids; TG, triglycerides; VLDL, very low-density lipoproteins

cardioprotective effects of estrogens has been attributed to the changes in LDL- and HDL-cholesterol. When lipoprotein subfractions are analyzed, a low risk profile is characterized by a low LDL-cholesterol and a raised HDL-cholesterol, particularly the HDL_2 subfraction, while the level of LDL-cholesterol is positively related to the risk of IHD[49].

Apolipoproteins are important for the transport of lipids and their uptake in peripheral tissues, and are important independent predictors of cardiovascular disease risk. Epidemiologic data have linked apolipoprotein B (ApoB) with cerebrovascular disease while ApoAI is inversely related to the risk. Lipoprotein(a) (Lp(a)) has been identified as an independent risk factor for atherosclerosis and coronary heart disease[50], although the underlying mechanism has not yet been clearly defined. Estrogen replacement treatment in postmenopausal women reduces Lp(a) levels[51]. An apparently beneficial effect of HRT on the risk of cardiovascular disease is probably mediated through a favorable effect on the lipid profile. In addition estrogen reduces central obesity, with a concomitant reduction in insulin levels. Indeed, current estrogen use may reduce the risk of type II diabetes mellitus by 20%[52].

Estrogen deficiency is associated with increases in levels of total cholesterol, LDL-cholesterol and Lp(a), and a reduction in HDL-cholesterol[53]; estrogen replacement reverses these changes. Progestins may increase the activity of hepatic lipoprotein lipase and therefore increase the catabolism of HDL_2, resulting in a lowering of the levels of HDL_2 and HDL-cholesterol[54]. In addition estrogen with cyclically administered progestogen has little or no effect on triglycerides[51]. When a progestogen was used in a continuous combined fashion along with estrogen, as an amenorrhea regimen, HDL levels were found to be reduced, however[55].

Changes in coagulation factors
The menopause results in changes in coagulation factors, with increases in fibrinogen[56], plasminogen activator inhibitor-1 (PAI-1)[57], factor VIIc[58] and antithrombin-III (AT-III)[59]. Estrogen replacement treatment is associated with increases in plasminogen, platelet count, factor VII, factor IX, factor X, factor XI, protein C and von Willebrand's factor, and with reductions in fibrinogen, AT-III, prothrombin time, tissue plasminogen activator, PAI-1, platelet aggregation time and protein S[60].

The interaction between these factors is also governed by a large buffering capacity to compensate, within limits for the effects of any derangement in an individual protein. Thus the predictive value of future occurrence of venous thrombosis as a result of estrogen replacement treatment, by measuring each individual clotting factor, is restricted to the finding of gross abnormalities only. Therefore one has to rely on the epidemiologic data, which have shown that there is a very small increase in the risk of venous thrombosis as a result of HRT use, an excess of 1 case in 5000 users[61,62]. These studies suggest that the risk of venous thromboembolism is greater during the first year, and that the risk then declines over the following 2 years and becomes not significantly different from controls after 3 years of use. Patients found to have protein S deficiency or activated protein C resistance such as those with factor V Leiden gene phenotype, require careful assessment of the risks and benefits of HRT, which have to be considered and tailored to the individual needs prior to embarking on treatment.

THE HERS STUDY

The Heart and Estrogen/Progestin Replacement Study (HERS) was a randomized placebo-controlled study of continuous combined conjugated estrogens (0.625 mg) plus 2.5 mg of medroxyprogesterone acetate (MPA) for the secondary prevention of IHD in women with an established diagnosis of IHD[63]. In contrast to the investigators' expectation there was an increase of IHD events in the treated group compared to the placebo group during the first two years of the study. However, when the data were processed to exclude IHD events during the first 2 years of the study, there was a trend towards a beneficial effect in the treated group[64]. This trial was a landmark in its field but unfortunately suffered from a number of pitfalls, which raised more questions than could be answered by it. The recruitment period was extended, with the majority of patients enrolled towards the end of the 18-month period, and the observation time was thus reduced to a mean of 4.1 as opposed to 4.75 years in the initial description of the protocol. Moreover the incidence of IHD events in the placebo group was 3.3%, which is significantly lower than the expected incidence of 5%. Such factors clearly undermine the statistical power of the study.

The study lacked an estrogen-only group and included only one type of progestin. The choice of the progestin and the duration of its administration might have been another factor in the results of the HERS report; MPA has been shown to affect adversely coronary arteries in monkeys[65,66]. The prothrombotic potential of women who experienced IHD events was not determined and in particular the genotyping for factor V Leiden; factor V Leiden mutation has also been linked to arterial disease[67].

CONCLUSION

It should be emphasized that the menopause is a positive step in a woman's life; it is the beginning of the post-reproductive phase of her life, when she may pursue a new career, education or vocation. The symptoms of estrogen deprivation can be relieved by estrogen treatment, which if taken long-term will help to prevent genital atrophy and reduce the risk of disabilities related to osteoporosis. There is increasing evidence for the role of HRT in reducing the risk of cardiovascular diseases and the incidence of colon cancer. These issues highlight the importance of HRT and rank it among the most significant preventative public health programs. The commitment to long-term HRT, however, is not an easy decision for women to make, especially when they are asymptomatic. In order to promote the acceptance of the preventative role of HRT in our aging society, the woman must be given the opportunity to ask questions after adequate counseling, and the balance of risks and benefits must be amply explained, such that she is enabled to make informed health choices.

ACKNOWLEDGEMENT

Sections of this chapter have previously been published in a review article (Al-Azzawi F. The menopause and its treatment in perspective. *Postgrad Med J* 2001;77:292–304).

REFERENCES

1. Kaplun A, ed. *Health Promotion and Chronic Illness: Discovering a New Quality of Health. European Series, No. 44*. WHO Regional Publications, 1992
2. MacNaughton J, Banah M, McCloud P, *et al*. Age related changes in follicle stimulating hormone, luteinizing hormone, oestradiol and immunoreactive inhibin in women of reproductive age. *Clin Endocrinol* 1992;36:339–45
3. Faddy MJ, Gosden RG, Gougeon A, *et al*. Accelerated disappearance of ovarian follicles in mid-life: implications for forecasting menopause. *Hum Reprod* 1992;7:1342–6
4. Faddy MJ, Gosden RG. A model conforming the decline in follicle numbers to the age of menopause in women. *Hum Reprod* 1996;11:1484–6
5. Taylor AH, Al-Azzawi F. Immunolocalisation of oestrogen receptor beta in human tissues. *J Mol Endocrinol* 2000;24:145–55
6. Bäckström T. Symptoms related to the menopause and sex steroid treatments. *Ciba Found Symp* 1995;191:171–80
7. Luine VN, McEwen BS. Effect of oestradiol on turnover of type A monoamine oxidase in brain. *J Neurochem* 1977;28:1221–7
8. Crowley WR. Effects of ovarian hormones on norepinephrine and dopamine turnover in individual hypothalamic and extrahypothalamic nuclei. *Neuroendocrinology* 1982;34:381–6
9. Paganini-Hill A, Henderson VW. Estrogen replacement therapy and risk of Alzheimer disease. *Arch Intern Med* 1996;156:2213–17
10. Yaffe K, Sawaya G, Lieberburg I, Grady D. Estrogen therapy in postmenopausal women: effects on cognitive function and dementia. *J Am Med Assoc* 1998;279:688–95
11. Maheux R, Naud F, Rioux M, *et al*. A randomized, double-blind, placebo-controlled study on the effect of conjugated estrogens on skin thickness. *Am J Obstet Gynecol* 1994;170:642–9
12. Ashcroft GS, Dodsworth J, van Boxtel E, *et al*. Estrogen accelerates cutaneous wound healing associated with an increase in TGF-beta1 levels. *Nature Med* 1997;3:1209–15

13. Cooper C. Femoral neck bone density and fracture risk. *Osteoporosis Int* 1996;6(Suppl 3):24–6

14. Riggs BL, Melton LJD. Involutional osteoporosis. *N Engl J Med* 1986;314:1676–86

15. Ott S. Bone density in adolescent. *N Engl J Med* 1991;325:1646–7

16. Wark JD. Osteoporosis: pathogenesis, diagnosis, prevention and management. In Urger HG, ed. *The Menopause: Clinical Endocrinology and Metabolism*. London: Baillière Tindall, 1993:151–81

17. Hui SL, Wiske PS, Norton J, Johnston CCJ. A prospective study of change in bone mass with age in postmenopausal women. *J Chron Dis* 1982;35:715–25

18. Marshall D, Johnell O, Wedel H. Meta-analysis of how well measures of bone mineral density predict occurrence of osteoporotic fractures. *Br Med J* 1996;312:1254–9

19. Galien R, Garcia T. Estrogen receptor impairs interleukin-6 expression by preventing protein binding on the NF-kappaB site. *Nucleic Acids Res* 1997;25:2424–9

20. Hughes DE, Dai A, Tiffee JC, *et al*. Estrogen promotes apoptosis of murine osteoclasts mediated by TGF-beta. *Nature Med* 1996;2:1132–6

21. Horowitz MC. Cytokines and estrogen in bone: anti-osteoporotic effects. *Science* 1993;260:626–7

22. Tiegs RD, Body JJ, Wahner HW, *et al*. Calcitonin secretion in postmenopausal osteoporosis. *N Engl J Med* 1985;312:1097–100

23. Chen C, Noland KA, Kalu DN. Modulation of intestinal vitamin D receptor by ovariectomy, estrogen and growth hormone. *Mech Ageing Dev* 1997;99:109–22

24. Colditz GA, Willett WC, Stampfer MJ, *et al*. Menopause and the risk of coronary heart disease in women. *N Engl J Med* 1987;316:1105–10

25. Stampfer MJ, Colditz GA. Estrogen replacement therapy and coronary heart disease: a quantitative assessment of the epidemiologic evidence. *Prev Med* 1991;20: 47–63

26. Grady D, Rubin SM, Petitti DB, *et al*. Hormone therapy to prevent disease and prolong life in postmenopausal women. *Ann Intern Med* 1992;117:1016–37

27. Voutilainen S, Hippeläinen M, Hulkko S, *et al*. Left ventricular diastolic function by Doppler echocardiography in relation to hormonal replacement therapy in healthy postmenopausal women. *Am J Cardiol* 1993;71:614–17

28. Pines A, Fisman E, Shemesh J, *et al*. Menopause-related changes in left ventricular function in healthy women. *Cardiology* 1992;80:413–16

29. Pines A, Fisman EZ, Levo Y, *et al*. Menopause-induced changes in left ventricular wall thickness. *Am J Cardiol* 1993;72:240–1

30. Villecco AS, de Aloysio D, de Liberali E, *et al*. High blood pressure and 'ischaemic' ECG patterns in climacteric women. *Maturitas* 1985;7:89–97

31. Staessen J, Bulpitt CJ, Fagard R, *et al*. The influence of menopause on blood pressure. *J Hum Hypertens* 1989;3:427–33

32. Botting R, Vane JR. Vasoactive mediators derived from the endothelium. *Arch Mal Coeur Vaiss* 1989;82:11–14

33. Collins P, Rosano GM, Jiang C, *et al*. Cardiovascular protection by oestrogen – a calcium antagonist effect? *Lancet* 1993;341:1264–5

34. Mugge A, Riedel M, Barton M, *et al*. Endothelium independent relaxation of human coronary arteries by 17 beta-oestradiol *in vitro*. *Cardiovasc Res* 1993;27:1939–42

35. Crane MG, Harris JJ, Winsor WD. Hypertension, oral contraceptive agents, and conjugated estrogens. *Ann Intern Med* 1971;74:13–21

36. Wren BG, Routledge DA. Blood pressure changes: oestrogens in climacteric women. *Med J Aust* 1981;2:528–31

37. Pfeffer RI, Kurosaki TT, Charlton SK. Estrogen use and blood pressure in later life. *Am J Epidemiol* 1979;110:469–78

38. Lip GY, Beevers M, Churchill D, Beevers DG. Hormone replacement therapy and blood pressure in hypertensive women. *J Hum Hypertens* 1994;8:491–4

39. Campbell S, Whitehead M. Oestrogen therapy and the menopausal syndrome. *Clin Obstet Gynaecol* 1977;4:31–47

40. Akkad AA, Halligan AW, Abrams K, Al-Azzawi F. Differing responses in blood pressure over 24 hours in normotensive women receiving oral or transdermal estrogen replacement therapy. *Obstet Gynecol* 1997;89:97–103

41. Pines A, Fisman EZ, Levo Y, *et al.* The effects of hormone replacement therapy in normal postmenopausal women: measurements of Doppler-derived parameters of aortic flow. *Am J Obstet Gynecol* 1991;164:806–12

42. Volterrani M, Rosano G, Coats A, *et al.* Estrogen acutely increases peripheral blood flow in postmenopausal women. *Am J Med* 1995;99:119–22

43. Gangar KF, Vyas S, Whitehead M, *et al.* Pulsatility index in internal carotid artery in relation to transdermal oestradiol and time since menopause. *Lancet* 1991;338:839–42

44. Rosano GM, Sarrel PM, Poole-Wilson PA, Collins P. Beneficial effect of oestrogen on exercise-induced myocardial ischaemia in women with coronary artery disease. *Lancet* 1993;342:133–6

45. Chester AH, Jiang C, Borland JA, *et al.* Oestrogen relaxes human epicardial coronary arteries through non-endothelium-dependent mechanisms. *Coron Artery Dis* 1995;6:417–22

46. Rodriguez G, Warkentin S, Risberg J, Rosadini G. Sex differences in regional cerebral blood flow. *J Cereb Blood Flow Metab* 1988;8:783–9

47. Penotti M, Nencioni T, Gabrielli L, *et al.* Blood flow variations in internal carotid and middle cerebral arteries induced by postmenopausal hormone replacement therapy. *Am J Obstet Gynecol* 1993;169:1226–32

48. Akkad A, Hartshorne T, Bell PR, Al-Azzawi F. Carotid plaque regression on oestrogen replacement: a pilot study. *Eur J Vasc Endovasc Surg* 1996;11:347–8

49. Thompson GR. The proving of the lipid hypothesis. *Curr Opin Lipidol* 1999;10:201–5

50. Scanu AM. Lipoprotein(a). A genetic risk factor for premature coronary heart disease. *J Am Med Assoc* 1992;267:3326–9

51. Nabulsi AA, Folsom AR, White A, *et al.* Association of hormone-replacement therapy with various cardiovascular risk factors in postmenopausal women. The Atherosclerosis Risk in Communities Study Investigators. *N Engl J Med* 1993;328:1069–75

52. Manson JE, Rimm EB, Colditz GA, *et al.* A prospective study of postmenopausal estrogen therapy and subsequent incidence of non-insulin-dependent diabetes mellitus. *Ann Epidemiol* 1992;2:665–73

53. Folsom AR, McGovern PG, Nabulsi AA, *et al.* Changes in plasma lipids and lipoproteins associated with starting or stopping postmenopausal hormone replacement therapy. Atherosclerosis Risk in Communities Study. *Am Heart J* 1996;132:952–8

54. Tikkanen MJ, Kuusi T, Nikkilä EA, Sipinen S. Post-menopausal hormone replacement therapy: effects of progestogens on serum lipids and lipoproteins. A review. *Maturitas* 1986;8:7–17

55. Al-Azzawi F, Wahab M, Habiba M, *et al.* Continuous combined hormone replacement therapy compared with tibolone. *Obstet Gynecol* 1999;93:258–64

56. Folsom AR, Wu KK, Davis CE, *et al.* Population correlates of plasma fibrinogen and factor VII, putative cardiovascular risk factors. *Atherosclerosis* 1991;91:191–205

57. Heinrich J, Sandkamp M, Kokott R, *et al.* Relationship of lipoprotein(a) to variables of coagulation and fibrinolysis in a healthy population. *Clin Chem* 1991;37:1950–4

58. Scarabin PY, Bonithon-Kopp C, Bara L, *et al.* Factor VII activation and menopausal status. *Thromb Res* 1990;57:227–34

59. Meade TW. Hormone replacement therapy and haemostatic function [published erratum appears in *Thromb Haemost* 1997;78:1304]. *Thromb Haemost* 1997;78:765–9

60. Low GDO. Coagulation, fibrinolysis and hormone replacement therapy. In Shaw RW, ed. *Oestrogen Deficiency: Causes and Consequences*. Carnforth, UK: Parthenon Publishing, 1996:29–44

61. Jick H, Derby LE, Myers MW, *et al.* Risk of hospital admission for idiopathic venous thromboembolism among users of postmenopausal oestrogens. *Lancet* 1996;348:981–3

62. Daly E, Vessey MP, Hawkins MM, *et al.* Risk of venous thromboembolism in users of hormone replacement therapy. *Lancet* 1996;348:977–80

63. Grady D, Applegate W, Bush T, *et al.* Heart and Estrogen/progestin Replacement Study (HERS): design, methods, and baseline characteristics. *Control Clin Trials* 1998;19:314–35

64. Hulley S, Grady D, Bush T, *et al.* Randomised trial of estrogen plus progestin for secondary prevention of coronary heart disease in postmenopausal women. *J Am Med Assoc* 1998;280:605–13

65. Adams MR, Register TC, Golden DL, *et al.* Medroxyprogesterone acetate antagonizes inhibitory effects of conjugated equine estrogens on coronary artery atherosclerosis. *Arterioscl Thromb Vasc Biol* 1997;17:217–21

66. Miyagawa K, Rösch J, Stanczyk F, Hermsmeyer K. Medroxyprogesterone interferes with ovarian steroid protection against coronary vasospasm. *Nature Med* 1997;3:324–7

67. Rosendaal FR, Siscovick DS, Schwartz SM, *et al.* A common prothrombin variant (20210 G to A) increases the risk of myocardial infarction in young women. *Blood* 1997;90:1747–50

2
Menstruation and methods of assessment of uterine bleeding

F. Al-Azzawi

INTRODUCTION

Menstruation (derived from the Latin 'mensis' or month) evolved in primates about 60 million years ago. It is generally accepted that it confers an evolutionary advantage, but the exact mechanism through which this advantage is achieved is not known. It may be that the provision of a newly developed endometrium potentially eligible to receive an implanting embryo adds a further layer to the species' reproductive selection process. Suggestions of a cleansing mechanism of potentially infected endometrial tissue[1] do not stand scrutiny when the commonly occurring retrograde menstruation, the existence of necrotic tissue within the uterus and the rich vascular spaces in the endometrial bed are considered. Over the last 150 years factors such as earlier menarche, smaller family size, the advent of effective contraceptive methods and bottle feeding have resulted in more frequent menstrual events. Whether a higher frequency of menstruation in itself results in an increased number of 'atypical cycles', or that changes in lifestyle constitute a major factor for increased menstrual complaints, is difficult to ascertain.

BLEEDING DURING THE MENSTRUAL CYCLE

Endometrial development represents a highly integrated cascade of events in response to cyclical ovarian function. Menstruation is an expression of the summation of preparatory events to a potential implantation that has not occurred in the previous cycle, and represents in itself the start of another series of preparative steps in response to the following ovarian cycle. As such, the occurrence of menstruation is perceived as evidence of potential fertility and health, and by the same token is a feature of the young female. Therefore menstruation is a significant event in women's lives and, irrespective of their sociocultural background, most women are clearly aware of their menstrual rhythm, especially the regularity of the event. Menses are more widely variable at both ends of reproductive life, but during the two decades of menstrual maturity (20–39 years of age) they tend to be much less variable.

Geographic location and ethnicity may play an important part in the pattern of menstruation. European women tend to have more bleeding/spotting days, while women from Latin America have shorter bleeding episodes and longer bleeding-free intervals. These features have been observed in those using oral contraceptive pills as well as in those menstruating spontaneously. Furthermore, only 25% of European women treated with depot medroxyprogesterone acetate (MPA) experienced amenorrhea by their fourth injection compared to 72% of women in North Africa[2]. However, there are no comparative data on the ethnicity or geographic location of menstrual events under the effect of hormone replacement therapy (HRT).

BLEEDING IN RESPONSE TO EXOGENOUS SEX STEROIDS

Premenopausal women

Exogenous sex steroid therapy is administered for various therapeutic indications, but primarily it is used for contraception and as HRT. The combined oral contraceptive pill is given either as a continuous estrogen–progestogen combination or in variable dose combinations in an attempt to mimic the ovarian cycle. The essence of the treatment is the provision of a minimal effective dose of estrogen (usually 30–35 µg of ethinylestradiol-containing pill) that overrides the level of endogenously produced estrogen, thus promoting suppression of follicle-stimulating hormone (FSH) and luteinizing hormone (LH). The concomitant administration of progestogen helps to down-regulate the expression of estrogen receptor, and enhances the degradation of estradiol within the endometrium, thus minimizing the endometrial growth stimulatory effect of estrogen, and renders the endometrium less suitable for implantation.

In perimenopausal women who complain of vasomotor symptoms while still menstruating, a state of relative estrogen deficiency can be assumed and therefore suppression of ovarian responses to gonadotropin can be achieved by lower doses of estrogen, for example 20 µg ethinylestradiol-containing pill. In the young as well as in the older premenopausal woman the respective doses of ethinylestradiol may not always be adequate to suppress the ovaries, allowing a spontaneous resurgence of endogenous sex steroid production, which leads to destabilization of the endometrium. This is clinically manifested as unscheduled bleeding, or break-through bleeding.

Increasing the dose of the progestogen may be adequate in some cases, but this is counterbalanced by a higher incidence of bloatedness, fluid retention and mastalgia. Furthermore, one should be mindful of the potential metabolic effect of long-term administration of high doses of progestogens, and therefore such regimens should be reviewed regularly. Alternatively a higher dose of ethinylestradiol (30 µg) may be required, but there is general concern about prescribing higher doses in older women. If abnormal uterine bleeding persists despite adjustments of treatment, the endometrial cavity should be fully investigated. Women in whom this occurs may have an endometrial polyp or submucous fibroids, and – particularly in the case of those with increased risk factors for developing endometrial neoplasia – should have an endometrial biopsy, preferably 4–6 weeks after the discontinuation of hormone treatment.

Changes in endometrial histology in response to the combined oral contraceptive pill are frequently described as 'retarded'[3], and similar descriptions have been applied to the endometria of postmenopausal women treated with HRT[4]. These descriptions may be justified in terms of poorer glandular development and stromal changes compared to the luteal phase endometrium of the natural cycle. However, the characteristics of metabolism and bioavailability of the acting steroids are different[5] and as such it is not unreasonable to assume that the mechanisms which lead to endometrial shedding may not be identical in the two situations. This issue is described in greater detail in Chapter 5.

Postmenopausal women

Cessation of menstruation – menopause – heralds a new role for the woman, free of the responsibility for reproduction. In some societies cessation of menstruation removes hurdles created by personal and social taboos restricting women from many activities and, therefore, this transition may be regarded positively by many. It enables the woman to pursue a career or vocation which was not available for her when she looked after the family.

The menopausal transition is marked by an estrogen deficiency state, regardless of whether symptoms of this state exist or not (Chapter 1). The benefits of estrogen replacement therapy in estrogen-deficient women have been widely documented. Such treatment relieves vasomotor symptoms, improves mental function, prevents bone loss and reduces the risk of cardiovascular disease. Administered to women with an intact uterus, unopposed estrogen may stimulate endometrial growth, and results in a high incidence of endometrial hyperplasia and a high risk of developing endometrial carcinoma[6,7], and may lead to a high incidence of gynecologic intervention[8]. It has been established that the administration of a progestogen for 10–12 days every 28 days may protect the endometrium against hyperplasia and may diminish the risk for developing endometrial carcinoma (see Chapter 7 for further details). It is interesting to note that sequential HRT regimens have been marketed as 28-day treatment cycles, when one might be able to argue for a calendar month-based cyclical progestogen administration. However, in the author's experience, a regimen designed to produce a 3-monthly bleeding pattern has not been widely successful, in view of the heavier bleeding episodes and the prevalence of progestogenic adverse effects due to the high dose of the progestogen used. Furthermore, endometrial hyperplasia at the end of the estrogen phase was detected in 15% of samples, although all were reversed after the progestogen phase[9]. Consequently, the long-term endometrial safety of such regimens remains to be ascertained.

The addition of progestogens in a cyclical manner results in the re-initiation of cyclical bleeding, and for the majority of postmenopausal women is not a welcome event. Re-initiation of menstrual discharge in postmenopausal women is regarded by the majority of women as a burden and serves little, if any, purpose. It is not surprising therefore that the induction of menstrual discharge becomes tolerable only as a price to be paid for the relief of symptoms. Consequently, in order to promote long-term continuation with postmenopausal HRT, the issue of regulation of menstrual episodes, in terms of cycle length, duration and amount of bleeding, becomes an essential 'bargaining tool'. Equally importantly, regulation enables the woman to predict the day of onset of bleeding in the following cycle, helps her to plan her life and increases her confidence in continuing with the treatment long-term.

The introduction of continuous combined estrogen–progestogen HRT (ccHRT) regimens is based on the premise that continuous progestogen administration down-regulates the estrogen receptor in the endometrium in a manner similar to the effect of the combined oral contraceptive pill, but given continuously rather than for 3 weeks out of 4. In this manner ccHRT is expected to induce a thin atrophic endometrium thereby achieving amenorrhea. The induction of an amenorrheic state is the most important feature for the increasing popularity of this type of HRT regimen. However, as many as 50% of women who commence ccHRT will experience bleeding episodes during the first 3–6 months, although for those who continue the treatment amenorrhea is achieved in over 90%, with a high continuation rate[10]. Other than the bleeding problems, women may discontinue ccHRT because of the adverse effects of progestogens. Long-term safety data are not available on other organ systems, for example the attenuation of bone sparing or cardiovascular benefits of estrogens.

One of the main pathophysiologic processes responsible for unscheduled bleeding in postmenopausal women on HRT is the bioavailability of the estrogen used. In particular, the susceptibility of estradiol for inactivation by 17β-dehydrogenase and subsequent metabolic clearance to the weaker estrone and its conjugates is higher than that of the resistant ethinylestradiol, or its 3-methyl ether. In addition sequential progestogens may be inadequate to sustain endometrial stability until the end of the progestogen phase.

Different progestogens have been used in combination with estrogen. Norethisterone (NET) is one of the most widely used progestogens in cyclical sequential regimens. However in 50% of instances withdrawal bleeding occurs before the end of the progestogen phase of treatment[11]. Early bleeders, defined as women who bleed before the end of the progestogen phase, experience episodes of withdrawal bleeding which are poorly predictable, prolonged and more heavy than in women whose withdrawal bleeding occurs after the end of the progestogen phase (Figure 2.1)[11]. Medroxyprogesterone acetate (MPA) has been used in preference to NET because of its lower androgenic adverse effect, but it has a less favorable bleeding pattern compared to other progestogens[12]. Women on MPA bleed earlier in the progestogen phase compared to those on levonorgestrel (LNG) or desogestrel[13,14]. It is not surprising, therefore, that these women are dissuaded from long-term HRT. The understanding of the bleeding phenomenon and the ability to predict which woman is likely to bleed irregularly may enhance the clinical management of these women and enable the clinician to adjust the HRT regimen appropriately[15]. It may also help to provide an opportunity for scientific evaluation of endometria that respond poorly to a particular HRT regimen.

At present the only tool available to us in evaluating the pattern of bleeding, in general, is data collection from the individual woman, and the only response to

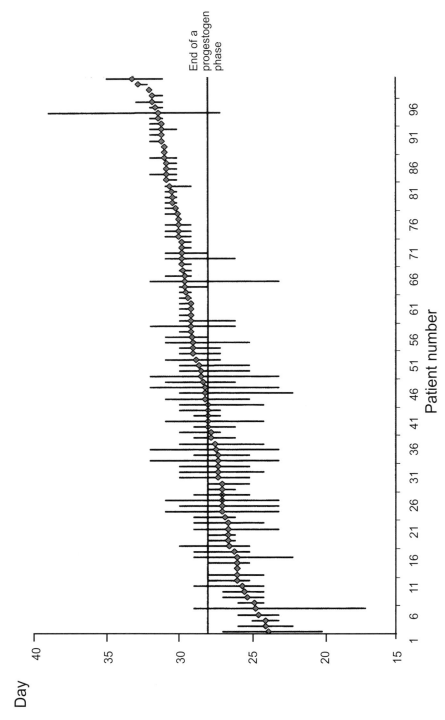

Figure 2.1. Mean day of onset of bleeding (± range) in women taking estradiol valerate 2 mg + cyclical norethisterone (NET) 1 mg. ©European Society of Human Reproduction and Embryology. Reproduced by permission of Oxford University Press/Human Reproduction, from Habiba MA, Bell SC, Abrams K, Al-Azzawi F. *Hum Reprod* 1996;11:503–8[11]

unsatisfactory bleeding pattern is to offer them a change in HRT regimen, which may induce more tolerable bleeding events.

METHODS OF ASSESSMENT OF THE MENSTRUAL EVENTS

Analysis of menstrual data may be based on the conventional perception of a 28-day menstrual cycle, which is useful when evaluating menstrual rhythm in conjunction with a 28-day sex steroid regimen. A reference period method of observation based on multiples of 30 days has been suggested[16], since menstruation occurs as a 'monthly event'. The reference period method is particularly useful when assessing bleeding events associated with intrauterine contraceptive device (IUCD) use, long-acting injectable contraceptive steroids, and with the progestogen-only pill – the minipill. This method assesses the bleeding events as they happen during the observation period. Regardless of the length of the reference period, be that a multiple of a 28-day cycle or 30 or 90 days, recording has to start with the commencement of treatment, which permits uniformity of assessment. Data obtained through the reference period method may not be easily assimilated in a clinical situation, particularly from the woman's viewpoint.

Many menstrual events will overlap the boundaries of the reference period. The number and percentage of those who do not bleed during the reference period should be reported separately and these data must be removed from the calculations of menstrual events within the reference period. Data derived from women who bleed throughout the reference period should be treated in a similar fashion. The World Health Organization (WHO) recommends the inclusion of these two different patterns of bleeding in the summary statistics and the counts of bleeding days. This issue is discussed in detail in Chapter 3.

Since the clinically important parameters of menstrual assessment are centered around the number of bleeding/spotting episodes, mean lengths of episodes and the range of lengths of bleeding-free intervals[17], it is proposed to evaluate the bleeding diaries using a reference period of 90 days, with the following parameters in mind:

(1) No bleeding: no days of bleeding/spotting entered throughout the reference period;

(2) Prolonged bleeding: bleeding/spotting episodes lasting 10 days or more during one reference period;

(3) Frequent bleeding: more than four bleeding/spotting episodes in one reference period;

(4) Infrequent bleeding: fewer than two bleeding/spotting episodes in one reference period; and

(5) Irregular bleeding: range of lengths of bleeding/spotting-free intervals not exceeding 17 days during one reference period.

A bleeding episode is defined as vaginal bleeding for 1 or more days with at least 2 bleed-free days before and after. A progestogen-associated bleed (PAB) means vaginal bleeding with any day of that episode starting between day 8 of progestogen administration of one cycle and day 7 after its discontinuation, inclusive; all other bleeding is defined as intermenstrual bleeding (IMB). The bleeding interval is the number of days between the first day of bleeding of two consecutive PABs.

In clinical studies involving postmenopausal women treated with a sequential combined HRT regimen, for example, the summary statistics of mean and standard deviation used for the description of the day of onset of bleeding, its duration and the amount of blood loss may give an idea as to the overall efficacy of that regimen. However, summary statistics tend to be dominated by data obtained from women with frequent short cycles. The problem of isolated episodes of bleeding between menses (IMB) and the problem of spotting events may complicate the summary statistics. Nevertheless, the omission of these events from the analysis may overlook salient factors for the discontinuation of treatment, and influence acceptability. Furthermore, such presentation of data ignores the individual woman's experience of the bleeding events. A method of analysis using the woman as the unit of analysis was first suggested in 1976[16]. In clinical practice we recommend the analysis of the individual woman's diary collected during a treatment phase in order to adjust the dose of treatment or mode of administration of HRT regimens[15]. A menstrual diary completed by an individual woman presents individual responses to a particular treatment and can be compared with the natural physiologic cycles, without forcing the data into an artificial method of analysis to which neither the woman nor the clinician is able to relate.

Data collection

Menstrual dates and patterns, as collected through interviews or questionnaires, are subject to problems of recall, and such data are less accurate the longer is the interval between the occurrence of the event and its reporting. Therefore, for more accurate data collection, prospective recording is favored and is best achieved by conscientious marking of bleeding episodes or spotting (blood loss that does not require sanitary protection) in a menstrual diary, as well as the marking of the bleed-free days. A bedtime-to-bedtime assessment interval is advised, or any other 24-hour interval, as long as it is consistent.

Regularity of the bleeding intervals

By repetition and reinforcement of the cycle concept, the regularity of menstruation has dominated the thoughts of women and of writers of medical literature, and for centuries had been linked to the lunar cycle. Towards the end of the 19th century clinical observations led to questioning the concept of regularity of menstruation, and in the first half of the 20th century numerous publications confirmed that in the general population both cycle length and duration of bleeding are variable – not only between women but between cycles in the individual woman as well. The published literature demonstrates that only 13–16% of the women studied had a range of cycle length (the difference between the longest and shortest cycle recorded) of less than 6 days. Furthermore, these studies show a steady decline in the average cycle length from the youngest to the oldest age groups, being lowest for women aged 25–39 and highest for 15–19-year-old women[18–22].

Studies on the menstrual pattern have involved collection of data over 1–2 years in most instances. Treloar and colleagues, however, reported on 2702 women from whom they collected annual diaries for an average duration of 9.6 years (maximum 29 years)[23]. In this study, and from other reports, there seems to be little justification for the concept of regularity of menstruation. These studies confirm the wide variability of the natural cycle in the individual woman, although the tendency for a less variable rhythm during menstrual maturity (ages 20–39) suggests the establishment of a more stable ovarian rhythm that controls menstruation.

The variation in cycle length is most probably related to the variable length of the follicular phase of the ovarian cycle since, following ovulation, the developmental milestones of the corpus luteum are rather constant. Nonetheless, in healthy women aberration of corpus luteum development and subsequent degeneration, albeit at a less variable rate, may in themselves be important factors in altering menstrual rhythm, pattern and duration of bleeding[24]. It is, therefore, prudent in a clinical sense to bear in mind these physiologic variations when assessing the complaints of menstrual irregularities and altered duration of menstrual loss. To evaluate the average length of the menstrual cycle a data set comprising a large number of menstrual-cycle lengths from a specified sample of women during a specified time interval is required. The data are pooled into one distribution with women contributing different cycle lengths to the pooled data. The mean and variance generated from this data set reflect the combined effect of within-woman and between-women variations.

Severity of bleeding

The amount of blood loss is difficult to document since the perceived amount of loss depends on a myriad factors related to personal hygiene and social and cultural attributes. A method for measurement of blood loss by alkaline elution of hematin from collected sanitary towels has been established. The improved accuracy of measurement of blood loss is countered by the laborious nature of the technique, which requires stringent precautions against transmission of blood-borne diseases and is certainly not practical for large-scale studies[25]. A surrogate measure was suggested by Higham and colleagues[26], based on a pictorial chart (Figure 2.2). The woman completes her menstrual diary on a daily basis, referring to the degree of soiling of sanitary towels or tampons. However, the reproducibility of this method has recently been questioned[27].

Intermenstrual bleeding

In analyzing menstrual diaries problems arise when trying to include episodes of spotting during the main menstrual phase, or the occurrence of truncated events – bleeding or spotting which occurs one or two days before or after the main menstrual event. Statistically presented summaries of menstrual data, particularly those collected over long observation periods, may not be seriously affected by such episodes in naturally menstruating women who are not using contraceptives. In these women they are largely accepted as part of the physiologic phenomenon.

CONCLUSION

The acceptability of exogenous sex steroid therapy for contraception or for HRT is affected by the withdrawal bleeding it creates. This involves regularity of day of onset, duration and severity of bleeding, and the occurrence of intermenstrual bleeding. In women using an IUCD, the oral contraceptive pill, or HRT such events may cause inconvenience or embarrassment, thus those women become

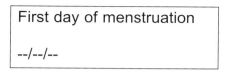

First day of menstruation

--/--/--

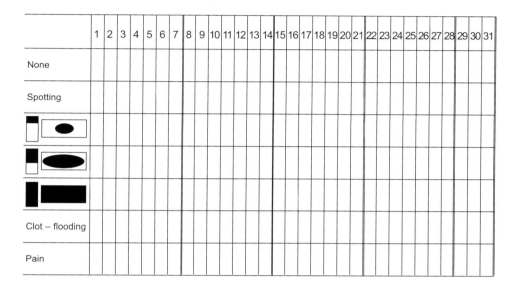

Figure 2.2. A pictorial menstrual calendar

more conscious of their occurrence. Therefore these events have to be included in such analyses in order to appreciate their extent. The occurrence of spotting, intermenstrual bleeding and truncated bleeding events may influence the acceptance of the treatment being administered. These issues become important for the postmenopausal woman undergoing hormonal treatment, where the exclusion of endometrial neoplasia is required. It frequently happens that an individualized approach to the pattern of bleeding is necessary, in order to enhance continuation of treatment. Many authors have tried to set up methods of assessing the regularity, length and duration of blood loss. All these methods, however, ignore the women's experience of the bleeding episodes. Analysis of the individual woman's diary to assess her bleeding pattern is the only way to address women's response to sex steroid treatment.

REFERENCES

1. Profet M. Menstruation as a defense against pathogens transported by sperm. *Q Rev Biol* 1993;68:335–86

2. Belsey EM, Peregoudov S. Determinants of menstrual bleeding patterns among women using natural and hormonal methods of contraception. I. Regional variations. *Contraception* 1988;38:227–42

3. Dallenbach-Hellweg G, Poulsen H, eds. *Histopathology of the Endometrium*. New York: Springer, 1996:105–9

4. Johannisson E, Brosens I, Cornillie F, *et al.* Morphometric study of the human endometrium following continuous exposure to levonorgestrel released from vaginal rings during 90 days. *Contraception* 1991;43:361–74

5. Goldzieher JW. Pharmacokinetics and metabolism of ethynyl estrogens. In Goldzieher JW, Fotherby K, eds. *Pharmacology of the Contraceptive Steroids*. New York: Raven, 1994: 127–53

6. Smith D, Prentice R, Thompson D, Herrman W. Association of exogenous estrogen and endometrial carcinoma. *N Engl J Med* 1975;293:1164–7

7. Weiss NS, Szekely DR, Austin DF. Increasing incidence of endometrial cancer in the United States. *N Engl J Med* 1976;294:1259–62

8. Ettinger B, Selby JV, Citron JT, *et al.* Gynecologic complications of cyclic estrogen progestin therapy. *Maturitas* 1993;17:197–204

9. Boerrigter PJ, van de Weijer PH, Baak JP, *et al.* Endometrial response in estrogen replacement therapy quarterly combined with a progestogen. *Maturitas* 1996;24:63–71

10. Doren M. Hormonal replacement regimens and bleeding. *Maturitas* 2000;34(Suppl):17–23

11. Habiba MA, Bell SC, Abrams K, Al-Azzawi F. Endometrial responses to hormone replacement therapy: the bleeding pattern. *Hum Reprod* 1996;11:503–8

12. Marslew U, Munk-Nielsen N, Nilas L, *et al.* Bleeding pattern and climacteric symptoms during different sequential combined HRT regimens in current use. *Maturitas* 1994; 19:225–37

13. Sporrong T, Rybo G, Mattsson LA, *et al.* An objective and subjective assessment of uterine blood loss in postmenopausal women on hormone replacement therapy. *Br J Obstet Gynaecol* 1992;99:399–401

14. Byrjalsen I, Thormann L, Meinecke B, *et al.* Sequential estrogen and progestogen therapy: assessment of progestational effects on the postmenopausal endometrium. *Obstet Gynecol* 1992;79:523–8

15. Al-Azzawi F, Wahab M, Thompson J, *et al.* Acceptability and patterns of uterine bleeding in sequential trimegestone-based hormone replacement therapy: a dose-ranging study. *Hum Reprod* 1999;14:636–41

16. Rodriguez G, Faundes-Latham A, Atkinson LE. An approach to the analysis of menstrual patterns in the critical evaluation of contraceptives. *Stud Fam Plann* 1976;7: 42–51

17. Belsey EM, Carlson N. The description of menstrual bleeding patterns: towards fewer measures. *Stat Med* 1991;10:267–84

18. Geist SH. The variability of menstrual rhythm and character. *Am J Obstet Gynecol* 1930; 20:320–3

19. Gunn DL, Jenkin PM, Gunn AL. Menstrual periodicity; statistical observations on a large sample of normal cases. *J Obstet Gynaecol Br Emp* 1937;44:839–79

20. Goldzieher J, Henkin A, Hamblen E, Durham N. Characteristics of the normal menstrual cycle. *Am J Obstet Gynecol* 1947;54:668–75

21. Matsumoto S, Nogami Y, Ohkuri S. Statistical studies on menstruation; a criticism on the definition of normal menstruation. *Gunma J Med Sci* 1962;11:294–318

22. Chiazze L, Brayer FT, Macisco JJ, *et al*. The length and variability of the human menstrual cycle. *J Am Med Assoc* 1968;203:377–80

23. Treloar A, Boynton R, Behn B, Brown B. Variation of the human menstrual cycle through reproductive life. *Int J Fertil* 1967;12:77–126

24. Wilcox AJ, Dunson D, Baird DD. The timing of the 'fertile window' in the menstrual cycle: day specific estimates from a prospective study. *Br Med J* 2000;321:1259–62

25. Hallberg L, Nilsson L. Constancy of individual menstrual blood loss. *Acta Obstet Gynecol Scand* 1964;43:352–9

26. Higham JM, O'Brien PM, Shaw RW. Assessment of menstrual blood loss using a pictorial chart. *Br J Obstet Gynaecol* 1990;97:734–9

27. Reid PC, Coker A, Coltart R. Assessment of menstrual blood loss using a pictorial chart: a validation study. *Br J Obstet Gynaecol* 2000;107:320–2

3
Analysis of menstrual bleeding diary data
J. R. Thompson

INTRODUCTION

The pattern of menstrual bleeding is often studied by asking women to complete a daily diary in which they note their bleeding days, perhaps also recording graded information on the amount of bleeding. Studies of this type need thoughtful design and careful analysis. Important design considerations include the length of the recording period and the points at which the recording should start and finish. A common approach is to use a fixed 'reference period', often taken to be 90 days, but it is also possible to use a fixed number of cycles or bleeding episodes[1]. When the data are analyzed, a decision must be made whether to reduce the data to a few summary measures or to find a method that models the full record. Whatever the approach the analysis must allow for both within-woman and between-women variation and it must be able to cope with the missing data that will almost certainly arise through either days when the diary is not filled in, or early drop-out from the study.

DESIGN OF THE STUDIES OF THE MENSTRUAL EVENTS

The decision concerning the most appropriate recording period will be influenced by practical considerations related to what it is possible to ask women to do, by the aims of the study and by considerations of statistical power. In treatment trials knowledge of the action of the drug might suggest a minimum treatment period, which should be long enough for the full impact of the treatment to become apparent and for any cumulative effects of the drug to be studied. Adverse events and drop-out owing to non-tolerance of a long-term treatment, such as oral contraception or hormone replacement therapy, may well only become apparent in long-term studies. Trials designed to look at population characteristics, such as average cycle length, will generally be more powerful if they recruit a large number of women for a relatively short time, while characteristics defined within women, such as cycle irregularity, will require longer records for each woman.

Where a treatment is taken for a fixed time, a specified number of treatment cycles might be used to define the length of the study. However, studies of untreated women are likely to be much more complex because of the difficulty of defining the natural cycle. The occurrence of breakthrough bleeding, spotting or missed periods can make it very difficult to define cycle length. It is this difficulty that has led many researchers to avoid talking of the natural cycle but instead to talk of bleeding-free intervals, and alongside this to adopt a reference period for the study. The length of the study can be chosen so that it is expected to include several bleeding episodes. The reference period method has two main drawbacks. First, it is likely that the study will end in the middle of a bleeding-free interval so that the woman's data would include an incomplete interval. To ignore such information would be inefficient while its inclusion will increase the complexity of the analysis. Second, the shorter is a woman's bleeding-free interval the more bleeding episodes she will contribute to the study. This opens the possibility that a naive analysis that does not distinguish between within-woman and between-women variability will be biased and underestimate the average bleeding-free interval of the population. This potential bias, sometimes called length-bias, will extend to other characteristics that are related to the length of the bleeding-free interval. Thus if the number of bleeding days is smaller when the bleeding-free interval is shorter, any method that biases the bleeding-free interval will also bias the number of bleeding days.

The design of any study should be made as efficient as possible by requiring the smallest number of women for the shortest time commensurate with answering the research questions. However there is also considerable advantage in a design that facilitates a simple analysis. The potential inefficiencies and biases of the reference period method can all be overcome, but at the expense of a complex analysis that is much more difficult to grasp than, say, a straightforward calculation of the average bleeding-free interval. It might well be wise to accept a little inefficiency in design if it makes the analysis simpler.

ANALYSIS

The most straightforward approach to analysis is to define a few summary measures that capture the features of the data that are of most interest to the researchers. Studies that have used multivariate data reduction techniques suggest that there are three main features of the pattern of bleeding, namely the time between bleeds, the amount of bleeding and the regularity of the pattern[2].

The freedom to devise a summary measure appropriate to a particular study has two drawbacks. First, there is a potential danger that the definition will be chosen to exaggerate the pattern that the researchers see in their data, and second, it may be difficult to compare with other studies in the literature or to combine studies in a meta-analysis. For these reasons it is advisable to adopt a common set of definitions whenever possible. Table 3.1 gives some definitions based on those developed by the World Health Organization (WHO)[3]. To use these definitions still requires a decision about what constitutes bleeding, in particular whether or not spotting is to be distinguished from bleeding.

Adopting the standard definitions given in Table 3.1 is likely to lead to a few slightly unsatisfactory diary summaries. For instance, the bleeding record that runs

$$\_\,\_\,\_\,\_\,\_\,X\_\,XXX\,\_\,\_$$

(where X represents a bleeding day and _ represents a bleeding-free day) will be interpreted as two bleeding episodes. Similarly, an isolated day of 'breakthrough bleeding' in the middle of a cycle will produce two segments, each about half the length of the natural cycle. It has been common practice for researchers to modify their definitions to try to accommodate such anomalies, but this is never entirely satisfactory, and whenever possible it would be better to adopt the standard definitions and then to compensate for any anomalies in the analysis. Thus the single bleeding day just before a longer bleeding segment suggests that it might be sensible to quote the average length of bleeding segments, and then the average if

Table 3.1. Standard definitions based on those developed by the World Health Organization

Bleeding episode	One or more consecutive days on which bleeding is noted in the diary bounded before and after by at least 1 bleeding-free day
Bleeding-free interval	One or more consecutive days on which bleeding is not noted in the diary bounded before and after by at least 1 bleeding day
Bleeding segment	A bleeding episode and the bleeding-free interval that immediately follows it

any very short segments are merged with the immediately following segment. The first figure provides a common standard against which other studies can be judged and the second figure, the average of very short segments merged with the immediately following segments, is equivalent to a modified definition. The use of the two figures has the added advantage that it acts as a sensitivity analysis showing the effect of isolated days on the average bleeding segment length.

The distorting effect of breakthrough bleeding on the average length of the bleeding segment and the associated effect of 'missed periods' might be overcome by changes in the definition of a bleeding segment, but once again it is better to tackle the problem by subsidiary analyses. The average of segments of lengths between, say, 15 and 40 days might be quoted alongside the average of all segments. In this case it will also be important to report the proportion of short and long segments.

Graphical presentation

It is unlikely that anyone will find a form of graphical presentation that adequately summarizes all aspects of a set of bleeding diaries. However the pattern of variation within and between women is neatly shown by a combination of the mean and range within women and a boxplot of the averages. Figure 3.1 illustrates such a plot using doses 1 and 4 from a dose-ranging study of trimegestone[4]. In the left-hand part of the plot the women are ordered according to their mean response, in this example their mean day of onset relative to the treatment cycle, and the means are plotted with vertical lines stretching between the minimum and maximum response for that woman. The right-hand side of the graph is a boxplot[5] of the mean responses of each woman and shows the between-women distribution for that dose. For the study illustrated in Figure 3.1 it can be seen that with the higher dose the distribution of the average response of most women becomes larger and much tighter, but that there are a few outliers, most with lower mean responses, and further that the within-woman variation is greater in those women.

The major feature omitted from Figure 3.1 is the degree of correlation between successive bleeding segments. From the point of view of developing a regression model to explain the response measurement in terms of explanatory variables such as drug treatment or the woman's age, it is important to know the size of any correlation and whether or not the amount of correlation decreases when bleeding segments of the same woman are further apart in time. Harlow and Zeger use a simple plot that shows the average correlation and the way that it changes when the time between segments increases[6]. Thus the first value is the correlation between

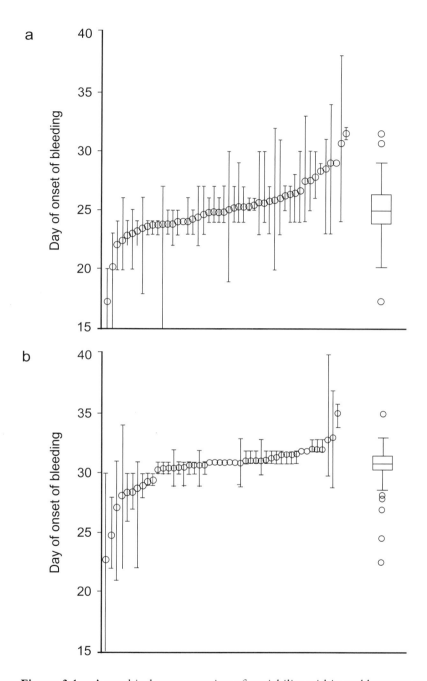

Figure 3.1. A graphical representation of variability within and between women from a dose-ranging study of trimegestone[4]. (**a**) Dose 1 (0.05 mg); (**b**) dose 2 (0.5 mg)

successive segments, the second point shows the correlation between segments that are one segment apart, and so on.

Numerical description of the variation within and between women

In the following section capital letters are used to denote characteristics of the population that are to be estimated, and lower case letters denote values calculated from the data.

Suppose that interest lies in the average segment length and that diaries are collected from a sample of n women. Each woman will have her own long-term average segment length T_i and by combining the data from several women the implicit concern is with trying to estimate the average segment length T for the population from which the women were sampled.

Let m_i represent the number of complete segments provided by the ith woman and t_{ij} be the observed segment length for the jth segment that she provides. The best way to summarize the data will depend on the precise definition of T. T might be thought of as the expected outcome from taking a woman at random and then observing the length of her next bleeding segment, i.e. the average of the T_i for this population.

The crude average of all of the data, t_{ij}, will systematically misrepresent T if the number of segments observed in a woman, m_i, is related to her individual average segment length T_i, such as when some women provide a lot of short segments and others a few long segments. When the m_i vary it will be safer to estimate the mean for each woman, $t_i = \Sigma t_{ij}/m_i$ and then to average those means $t = \Sigma t_i/n$.

Just as important as the bias that might arise is the question of the accuracy of the resulting sample mean, for this will influence the calculation of confidence intervals and any hypothesis tests. Suppose that the ith woman has segments that vary in length with a true variance of V_i, and the true means for each of the women, T_i, vary across our population with a between-women variance V. Estimates of the within-woman variance V_i will give results which will be inaccurate if the number of segments on that woman is small, in which case it may be better to average the V_i across all of the women and get an average within-woman variance which will be more stable.

Estimating the between-women variance presents an extra problem. Ideally the calculation should take the variance of the true means, T_i, but these are not available so it is natural to take the variance of the observed means, t_i, instead.

However, because the observed means are subject to within-woman variability the variance of the t_i will tend to overestimate the true between-women variance. Adjustment is simply to subtract the uncertainty in the observed means, t_i. That is:

variance between women = variance (t_i) – variance within women / m*

where m* can be taken as the average number of cycles per woman. Snedecor and Cochran[7] give a more accurate formula for use when the numbers of cycles per woman differ but it gives virtually the same result as taking the average number of cycles. A convenient way to obtain estimates of within-woman and between-women variability is to derive them from the output of an analysis of variance table. Snedecor and Cochran describe how to do this[7].

For dose 1 shown in Figure 3.1 the average within-woman variance is 5.97 days^2 and the variance between women is 3.83 days^2, showing that the within-woman variation is a little more important than the variation between women. For the other dose shown in Figure 3.1 the corresponding variances are 3.68 days^2 and 2.70 days^2. Again the within-woman variation is slightly greater than the between-women variation but the increased dose has reduced both types of variation.

Providing that consecutive segment lengths are independent, the variance of the mean that is calculated from the data on the ith woman will have a variance V_i/m_i. The average across women, t, will have a variance equal to

$$1/n(V + I/n\Sigma V_i/m_i)$$

That is, the accuracy of the mean, t, will depend on both the within-woman variability, V_i, and the between-women variability, V, and this will be estimated by substituting data-based values in place of the population variances often under the assumption that the within-woman variance, V_i, is the same for each woman. The square root of the estimated variance is the standard error (SE) of t and can be used to calculate approximate 95% confidence intervals based on t ± 2 SE.

The form of the formula for the standard error can help us to design an efficient study. If the variability in segment length within a woman, V_i, is large then increasing m_i, the number of bleeding segments observed for that woman, will reduce the size of the standard error. Conversely, if it is the variability between women, V, that is large then it will be sensible to increase n, the number of women in the study. Power calculations that are used to arrive at the minimum sample size for a study designed to test a particular hypothesis will require a prior guess at the likely sizes of V and V_i so that an anticipated standard error can be calculated.

The formula for the variance of t is based on the assumption that the data are independent. In terms of the between-women variability, this assumes that the women are a representative (ideally random) sample from the population under study. In terms of the within-woman variability, this assumes that consecutive segment lengths are independent; that is, when a woman has an unusually short segment she is not more likely to follow this by a second short segment or an unusually long segment. The patterns that could occur in successive segments are numerous and varied but a simple investigation of them might be made in terms of the correlation, R_i, between segment values for the ith woman that are successive, one segment apart, two segments apart, etc., as described above when discussing graphical presentation. These correlations should be estimated for each woman. If the number of segments m_i is small then the estimated within-woman correlations will not be very accurate and when there is no reason to suppose that some women show more correlation than others it will be sensible to average the correlations across the women. If the correlations R_i remain the same regardless of the interval between the segments then the variance of an individual woman's mean t_i will not be V_i/m_i but rather

$$V_i/m_i \, (1 + (m_i - 1)R_i)$$

so that if R_i is large and positive the accuracy of the mean t_i as an estimate of that woman's true mean T_i can be seriously reduced.

When these numerical summaries are calculated for the data shown in Figure 3.1 we obtain the results shown in Table 3.2. The standard error of the mean for dose 1 is thus 0.30 and for the higher dose is 0.26. The difference between the means for the two doses is 5.48 and its standard error is $\sqrt{0.3^2 + 0.26^2} = 0.40$. In this data set there is a slight tendency for short segments to follow longer ones with an average correlation between consecutive segments of -0.13. Allowing for this reduces the standard error slightly to 0.38.

Table 3.2. Calculations for the trimegestone data illustrated in Figure 3.1

	Number of women (n)	Mean (t)	Average within-woman variance	Between-women variance
Dose 1	60	25.18	5.97	3.83
Dose 4	57	30.66	3.68	2.70

Similar calculations were used by Harlow and Zeger for the analysis of menstrual diary data for untreated women[6]. They analyzed segments between 17 and 43 days in length and found the average within-woman variance (v_i) to be 13.5 days^2 and the between-women variance (v) to be 7.4 days^2. They further found that the average correlation between segment lengths for the same woman (r_i) was approximately 0.3 and the degree of correlation did not vary greatly with the interval between the segments. As their analysis was restricted to segments between 17 and 43 days in length they had to be careful when investigating the effect of a treatment or exposure on segment length. For instance the impact of stress might be to change the average segment length and also to increase the frequency of segments outside the 17–43-day window. They addressed this by using two models, one of the average length and another of the proportion of long segments.

Regression modeling

A regression model is a summary of the relationship between a feature of the bleeding, such as bleeding segment length, and explanatory variables. The explanatory variables are potentially of three types: features that are, for a particular woman, constant over the whole study, features that are constant over each segment and features that vary from day to day. If day-to-day variation is important then the records for individual days will need to be modeled and it will not make sense to try to model summary statistics such as the bleeding segment length. In practice it is much more likely that the important explanatory variables will be constant over the study or only vary between segments. For instance, Murphy and colleagues investigated the effect of body mass index (BMI) on segment length using the BMI measured at the start of each segment[8].

One regression model of interest in the comparison of the two doses of trimegestone would relate the day of onset of bleeding to the dose and the cycle number. Such a model would simultaneously quantify the effect of dose and investigate whether the day of onset tended to become later as the trial progressed. Using the usual notation for a regression such a model might be written as

$$\mu_{ij} = \beta_0 + \beta_1 \text{ dose} + \beta_2 \text{ cycle number}$$

where μ_{ij} is the predicted day of onset for woman i in cycle j and the coefficients β_0, β_1 and β_2 are the unknown values that are to be estimated. To complete the regression and facilitate the estimate of the coefficients it is necessary to specify how the observations y_{ij} will vary about this predicted value μ_{ij}. In general the form of a regression model for the response y_{ij} of the ith woman in her jth cycle sets up a relationship between the parameters of the distribution of y and a set of K explanatory variables x_{ijk}, $k = 1 \dots K$. The most commonly used model assumes that the measurements are normally distributed with constant variance and a mean that depends linearly on the explanatory variables. Written concisely, that is,

$$y_{ij} \sim N(\mu_{ij}, \sigma^2)$$

and

$$\mu_{ij} = \Sigma \beta_k x_{ijk}$$

Typically the responses y_{ij} might be measurements of segment length or amount of bleeding and the explanatory variables x_{ijk} might be measurements of treatment, age, smoking or stress.

This multiple regression model assumes that cycles in the same woman are no more similar than cycles from different women who share the same explanatory variables; that is, it does not distinguish between within-woman and between-women variability. This is unlikely to be a good representation of the data in examples such as the trimegestone study, in which case the model can be modified to include a subject term α_i which measures the characteristics of the ith woman that are not captured by the measured explanatory variables. Then the expression for the average response becomes

$$\mu_{ij} = \alpha_i + \Sigma \beta_k x_{ijk}$$

Unless the amount of data on each woman is very large it is not a good idea to fit this model by multiple regression because the resulting estimates are not very reliable. It is much better to assume a distribution for the α_i and to fit the model as a mixed linear regression. This is the approach adopted by Harlow and Zeger[6] and Al-Azzawi and colleagues[4]. It implicitly assumes equal correlation between pairs of responses for the same woman no matter how far apart the segments are in time.

Using modern statistical packages the form of the model that is finally adopted can incorporate any number of refinements. The variance σ^2 might also depend on the explanatory variables, the distribution might not be normal, the response might not depend linearly on the explanatory variables, or perhaps the degree of correlation between segments decreases with the time between them. For the purpose of interpreting the model, interest usually lies in the size of the coefficients β_k, which tell us how the explanatory variables affect the response. Typically these coefficients do not vary greatly as the variance structure of the regression model is

Table 3.3. Three regression models fitted to the trimegestone data illustrated in Figure 3.1

	Regression (SE)	Mixed model (SE)	GEE (SE)
Constant	25.03 (0.31)	25.18 (0.28)	25.03 (0.27)
Dose	5.49 (0.26)	5.47 (0.40)	5.49 (0.37)
Cycle number	0.05 (0.08)	0.04 (0.06)	0.05 (0.05)

GEE, generalized estimating equations; SE, standard error

refined although the standard errors of β_k may change quite dramatically, usually showing that models that are too simplistic exaggerate the accuracy with which the coefficients can be estimated and consequently make explanatory variables appear more significant than they actually are. Deciding when a model is adequate requires experience and judgement for there is no automatic procedure for determining the best model.

To illustrate the impact of refining the regression, the data on the two doses depicted in Figure 3.1 have been modeled. Initially it was supposed that the day of onset was normally distributed with constant variance and a mean,

$$\mu_{ij} = \beta_0 + \beta_1 \text{ dose} + \beta_2 \text{ cycle number}$$

This allows for a difference between doses and for an effect that increases steadily throughout the trial. The results are shown in the first column of Table 3.3. In the second analysis a subject term α_i is added to the model and fitted as a mixed model. The results are shown in the second column of Table 3.3. In the third analysis the dependence on the assumption of normality is weakened and a technique known as generalized estimating equations (GEE) is used to fit the model. All three models were fitted using the statistical package Genstat[9].

The adjustment for cycle number is very small and so the constant in Table 3.3 approximately equals the mean for dose 1, which was calculated previously using summary statistics to be 25.18 (standard error (SE) = 0.30) and the dose effect in Table 3.3 is the difference between doses that was previously estimated to be 5.48

(SE = 0.40). The calculation of means and standard errors as summarized in Table 3.2 allows for between-women and within-woman variation and is similar in approach to the mixed model or the GEE. For this study the next refinement might be to allow the variance to vary with dose as well as the means. The simple regression model does not represent the variability very well and overestimates the precision of the trial. Independent multiple regression is best avoided when analyzing diary data, but there is unlikely to be much to choose between the many models that allow for within-subject correlation in response.

CONCLUSION

The main recommendations for the analysis of menstrual diary data are that whenever possible standard definitions of a bleeding segment should be employed to facilitate comparison between studies, and that it is essential that the analysis incorporates both within-woman and between-women variability. Figure 3.1 shows how a single plot can be used to illustrate both types of variation and the section on the numerical description of the variation shows how the types of variation can be quantified. Failure to distinguish between within-woman and between-women variability will cause the analysis to give a falsely optimistic impression of the accuracy of the study. When several explanatory variables are to be incorporated into the analysis a regression model should be used. However the regression also needs to distinguish between within-woman and between-women variability or it too will exaggerate the precision of the study.

REFERENCES

1. Rodriguez G, Faundes-Latham A, Atkinson LE. An approach to the analysis of menstrual patterns in the critical evaluation of contraceptives. *Stud Fam Plann* 1976;7:42–51
2. Belsey EM, Carlson N. The description of menstrual bleeding patterns: towards fewer measures. *Stat Med* 1991;10:267–84
3. Belsey EM, Farley TMM. The analysis of menstrual bleeding patterns: a review. *Appl Stochastic Models Data Anal* 1987;3:151–60
4. Al-Azzawi F, Wahab M, Thompson J, *et al*. Acceptability and patterns of uterine bleeding in sequential trimegestone-based hormone replacement therapy: a dose-ranging study. *Hum Reprod* 1999;14:636–41
5. Cleveland W. *Visualizing Data*. Summit, NJ: Hobart Press, 1993
6. Harlow SD, Zeger SL. An application of longitudinal methods to the analysis of menstrual diary data. *J Clin Epidemiol* 1991;44:1015–25

7. Snedecor G, Cochran W. In *Statistical Methods*, 6th edn. Ames, Iowa: Iowa State University Press, 1978

8. Murphy SA, Bentley GR, O'Hanesian MA. An analysis for menstrual data with time-varying covariates. *Stat Med* 1995;14:1843–57

9. Genstat. *Genstat 5 Committee, GENSTAT 5 Release 3 References Manual*. Oxford: Clarenden, 1993

4
Action of sex steroid hormones
A. H. Taylor

INTRODUCTION

Steroids are commonly employed in current clinical practice; estrogens alone or in combination with progestogens as hormone replacement therapy (HRT) are used to ameliorate the symptoms of the menopause[1–4], cardiovascular morbidity and mortality[5], and osteoporosis[6]. Estrogens also delay the onset of Alzheimer's disease[7], with some suggestion that familial Alzheimer's disease may be prevented[8]. Estrogens in combination with progestogens or progestogens alone are well-established contraceptives[9], and anti-progesterones are used for the termination of pregnancy[10,11]. Finally, anti-estrogens are commonly employed in the prevention and treatment of breast cancer[12,13].

The benefits of these steroids are, however, limited by their adverse side-effects, which lead to disorders in endometrial function including inappropriate bleeding, endometrial proliferation, hyperplasia and sometimes malignancy during HRT and anti-estrogen treatment or menstrual dysfunction during HRT and oral contraception. The reason for steroid-induced endometrial disordering is poorly understood, but recent advances in studies that investigate steroid hormone action at the molecular level are providing important clues that might help clinicians and scientists to provide better treatments for symptoms of the menopause. Chief among these discoveries is the presence of a novel estrogen receptor and a clearer understanding of estrogen and progesterone action in many classical and non-classical target tissues. It is also clear that the two estrogen receptors (ER) and the progesterone receptor (PR) genes are themselves regulated by estrogen. Additionally, steroids also regulate the accessory molecules necessary for efficient steroid receptor function. There is increasing evidence that functionally distinct PR isoforms, PR_A and PR_B, are differentially expressed in the endometrium and breast, leading to the notion that these and other steroid receptor isoforms may also be differentially expressed in other target tissues. Therefore, the ratio of different ER or PR isoforms may cause some of the tissue-specific and adverse effects of steroid hormones in the endometrium.

This review of the literature describes the 'key players' in steroid hormone action with the postmenopausal woman in mind. How sex steroid hormones regulate the expression of ER and PR isoforms is presented and a brief mechanism of action for these receptors is given. For a more detailed and comprehensive review of anti-estrogen and anti-progesterone receptor action, the reader is directed to recent reviews[11,13–15].

ESTROGEN AND PROGESTERONE RECEPTORS

ER and PR belong to the steroid hormone receptor family of nuclear hormone receptors that are a subset of the thyroid hormone/steroid hormone receptor superfamily of nuclear receptor transcription factors[16]. The superfamily that includes estrogen, progesterone, mineralocorticoid, glucocorticoid, vitamin D, retinoic and thyroid hormone receptors has features common to all family members. All the above receptors are modular proteins that have had functional regions assigned to individual domains with specific functions (Figure 4.1)[17]. There are five distinct regions in all steroid hormone receptors, termed A/B; C; D; E and for the estrogen receptor family there is an additional region termed F (Figure 4.1). The N-terminal A/B region contains a cell- and promoter-specific transactivating function (often called TAF-1 but more commonly called AF-1) that can be activated in the absence of ligand[18]. The C region, which contains the DNA-binding domain, has crucial amino acid sequences that create the two zinc fingers that make direct contact with chromatin sequences. This region also contains other important functions in addition to the DNA-binding domain, since it has phosphorylation sites[19] and the dimerization domain[16]. The D region is called the hinge domain, because during receptor activation by ligand a conformational change occurs in this region of the molecule that is thought simultaneously to expose the nuclear localization signal[16] and the dimerization domain[20]. Finally the C-terminal region of steroid receptors contains the ligand-binding domain (LBD); in the estrogen receptor this region is called E/F, and in the progesterone receptor the F region is missing (Figure 4.2). The E region in both types of receptor binds the respective ligand that gives the receptor its name and confers ligand-dependent specificity on the molecule. What role the F region plays in ER action is still under debate, but the consensus of opinion is that it plays a role in the stabilization of the receptor–DNA complex to modulate the level of transcription induced by agonist-occupied ER[21,22]. Within the E region are the ligand-dependent transactivation function (AF-2) and the second dimerization domain, which allows the formation of ER–ER dimers[23].

Estrogen receptor subtypes

The classic ER (now called ERα) is a protein of 595 amino acids and has a relative molecular mass of ~66 kDa[24]. The second ER, called ERβ, is a smaller protein consisting of 485 amino acids with a relative molecular mass of ~54–55 kDa[25,26]. There is significant homology between these two receptor subtypes, especially in the DNA-binding domain (DBD) (96%) and in the LBD (53%) but not elsewhere in the molecules (Figure 4.1)[27]. The lower level of homology in the LBD originally suggested that the ERβ receptor might have a different specificity for estrogen binding compared to ERα[28]. *In vitro* experiments have shown that the affinities of these two receptors are similar but not identical, with K_d values in the single and tens of nmol/l range for ERα and ERβ, respectively[29–31]. It has been suggested that these data are the reason for some of the tissue-specific effects of some selective estrogen receptor modulators (SERMs)[32,33]. However, this is not the entire story for ER subtypes. Recently an ERγ has been postulated[34] because of the presence of estrogenic activity in the double ER knockout mouse (called DERKO mouse), and a non-ERα/non-ERβ isoform has been found in the brain of the goldfish[35]. This molecule is much larger than either ERα or ERβ, is located on a different chromosome to either ERα or ERβ and is confined solely to the goldfish brain. Mammalian brains also make a high molecular weight ER that reacts with some ERα antibodies[36]. Could this be mammalian ERγ?

Another discovery was of a novel androgen receptor from a Japanese eel cDNA library[37] that has high affinity for estrogens and that is postulated to be another ER isoform, which is generated from a gene found on a different chromosome to ERα, ERβ or ERγ[37]. These data suggest that other forms of the ER (ERγ or ERδ?) might exist in the human that could attenuate or modulate the action of estrogen in some tissues. There is no doubt that truncated and alternatively spliced isoforms of the ERα and ERβ proteins are produced and have important regulatory functions that may be related to disease[38]. For example, truncated ERα proteins, both experimentally and *in vivo*, act as dominant repressive agents to inhibit estrogen action in the breast and other tissues[39,40]. Indeed, ERβ binds tamoxifen (a SERM) with the same affinity as ERα, but in transient transfection studies does not show the agonist

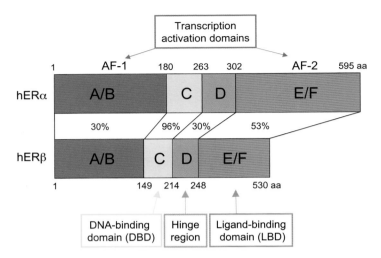

Figure 4.1. Structural comparison of human estrogen receptors (ERs) ERα and ERβ. Regions A–F represent the classical nomenclature for structurally similar amino acid (aa) sequences. Amino acid sequence numbers from the N-terminal are written on each bar, representing the mature ER protein molecule, and the percentage homology between the two proteins is presented. Key functional elements and regions are shown, including the transcription activation domains AF-1 and AF-2. The figure is drawn to emphasize the different sizes of the two receptor protein molecules

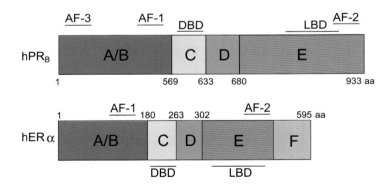

Figure 4.2. Structural comparison of human estrogen receptor (ERα) with progesterone receptor (PR$_B$). Regions A–F of the ERα protein are the same as those in Figure 4.1. The structure of the human PR is similar to that of ERα in that both molecules contain ligand-binding domains (LBD) specific for the hormone each protein binds. Both proteins also contain specific DNA-binding domains (DBD), transcription activation domains (AF-1 in the A/B region and AF-2 in the E region). The PR$_B$ receptor has an additional transcription activation domain (AF-3) in the A/B region which is not present in either ER isoform or the alternative PR, PR$_A$. Both PR proteins are significantly larger than ERα or ERβ. aa, amino acid

function that ERα does in the same system[41]. Indeed, more up-to-date data suggest that tamoxifen and perhaps other SERMs (such as raloxifene) may modulate gene transcription via interaction with the ERβ protein, which in turn binds directly to AP-1 proteins bound to its response element[42,43], but these data need to be confirmed. However, the data also suggest that some estrogens may have different actions in different tissues dependent on ER subtype expression and that alternative estrogen actions depend upon differential ER isoform expression[41].

Progesterone receptor subtypes

The PR also exists in two distinct isoforms[44], termed PR_A (~94 kDa) and PR_B (~114 kDa). Unlike the estrogen receptors, the two PRs are generated from the same gene by alternative transcription from two distinct promoters (Figure 4.3). Both receptors bind progestogens in a similar manner, with equivalent binding affinities to both ligand and DNA, but show different

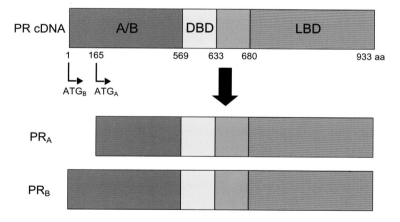

Figure 4.3. Progesterone receptor (PR) isoforms are generated from the same DNA sequence. Each of the PR isoforms PR_A and PR_B is generated from the same gene by alternative transcriptional initiation. The PR_B protein is generated from the upstream transcriptional start site (ATG_B), whereas PR_A is generated from a proximal transcriptional start site (ATG_A). The two receptors thus have different promoter sequences and consequently different expression patterns. The PR_A protein is 164 amino acids (aa) shorter than PR_B, with relative masses of ~94 kDa and ~114 kDa, respectively

functional activities in a cell type-, promoter- or ligand-specific manner[45,46]. Both PR isoforms are generated in both the endometrium and the breast, and recent data suggest that there are changes in the ratio of PR_A to PR_B during the menstrual cycle[47]. This opens the possibility that $PR_A:PR_B$ ratios that are important in controlling normal menstrual function are perturbed in the menopause owing either to inappropriate expression or to loss of expression of the appropriate PR receptor.

ER and PR tissue distribution

Owing to the roles of estrogen and progestogens in the control of sexual function, it is not surprising to find ERs and PRs in reproductive tissues and higher centers in the central nervous system that are involved in reproduction[48-50]. However, ERs and PRs are also expressed in non-reproductive tissues. The endothelium is a good example of a tissue that contains and expresses all four receptor types discussed in this review[51]. Although it is known that estrogens prevent intimal hyperplasia through activation of the ERβ-dependent pathway[52], the exact roles of ERα receptors and PRs in the regulation of endothelial cell function are poorly understood. The receptors are also found in other sites important to the understanding of postmenopausal pathology, such as the bone and brain[53-55]. Although it has been appreciated that ERα is present and important in osteoblasts and osteoclasts, it has only recently been realized that ERβ also plays an important role in maintaining bone mineral density[54]. Recently PRs were also found in bone cells where they attenuate the actions of estrogen on bone mineral density, thereby potentially weakening bone and accelerating osteoporosis in some individuals[56].

There also seems to be differential expression of ERα and ERβ isoforms in the human brain[57]. Some of the estrogenic effects of HRT are directly implicated in the brain, because postmenopausal complaints of headache, stress, confusion and 'word loss' symptoms are all ameliorated with HRT[58]. In addition HRT is also thought to delay or even prevent the onset of Alzheimer's disease, although any potential mechanism is presumably through the prevention of senile plaque production. Indeed, recent evidence has co-localized the lack of ERβ expression with sites of presenilin-1 expression[7]. Presenilin-1 is a proteolytic enzyme that converts amyloid precursor protein to amyloid-β peptide, the main insoluble protein found in senile plaques[59]. The suggestion is that some individuals lose the ability to control presenilin-1 expression, which leads to amyloid-β peptide deposition. The lack of control of presenilin-1 expression could be due to loss of ERβ expression at the site of deposition or through an unrelated mechanism involving ERα[60]. Of course, these hypotheses require testing and the data generated thus far need confirming, but it is encouraging to believe that understanding the etiology of Alzheimer's disease and, it is hoped, a potential cure are only a few years away.

ER and PR expression in the endometrium through the menstrual cycle

Changes in cyclical sex steroid levels are associated with well-described fluctuations of their respective receptors in the endometrium and breast, but not in other tissues[61–63]. Both ER isoforms appear to increase to a maximal expression in the proliferative phase of the cycle and decline in both the glandular and stromal compartments in the secretory phases[64]. However, there has not yet been a definitive study on the expression of ERβ protein in the endometrium of the normal woman. Previous data have only been generated from mRNA studies[65], which could be misleading, in as much as the levels of functional protein do not always reflect mRNA concentrations. In many tissues ERβ protein seems to disappear when the tissue is actively dividing, causing some researchers to conclude that ERβ acts as an anti-proliferative molecule[66]. If this is correct, then it might explain the adverse effects seen with some estrogen preparations and SERMs, since the premise would be that such molecules would preferentially and differentially activate ERα-dependent gene transcription. However, in general ER isoform expression appears to be up-regulated by 17β-estradiol, and autologous up-regulation of ERα is attenuated by progesterone during the menstrual cycle. The molecular mechanisms underlying these observations are not understood, but must involve interactions between ER and PR, perhaps through an intermediary protein. Interestingly, this effect appears to be tissue- or cell-specific, because the autologous up-regulation seen in endometrial cells is seen as autologous down-regulation in the liver, endothelial cells and the breast[67,68]. This interesting feature of steroid receptor regulation needs much more investigation, but suggests that the molecular mechanisms involved are likely to differ between tissues studied, and a general, all tissue-encompassing mechanism is unlikely.

The expression of uterine PR is principally regulated by estrogen via ERα, although it is not known what role ERβ plays in this process. Estrogen appears to up-regulate PR expression at the transcriptional level, even though there does not appear to be a consensus estrogen response element (ERE) in the PR promoter[69,70]. A pre-ovulatory surge of estrogen or exogenous estrogen administration[71] up-regulates both PR_A and PR_B, and progesterone has no effect on the endometrium in the absence of estrogen priming, owing to the lack of PR expression[72]. Progesterone has an anti-PR effect by decreasing ER levels and by direct interaction with its own receptor degradation via increased receptor turnover[63]. However, PRs are also regulated by other mechanisms in the endometrium. Recent studies with the ERα and ERβ knockout mice (ERKO and BERKO, respectively) have shown that PR expression still occurs in the presence of endogenous estrogen, which suggests that both ERs are involved in uterine PR expression[73]. In the endometrium, the PR_B receptor is the more active molecule and is regulated more strongly by estrogen than PR_A[74,75]. Accordingly, PR_B down-regulates PR_B but not PR_A expression, whereas PR_A is a strong inhibitor of both PR_A and PR_B expression[76,77]. This suggests that the ratio of PR_A to PR_B in any particular cell type could dictate the phenotype of that cell. Recent data suggest that this notion is correct. PR_A is less sensitive to hormonal fluctuations and so is expressed at a higher concentration in endometrial stromal cells compared to either PR_B or PR_A expression in glandular epithelial cells[63] during the progesterone-dependent luteal phase. This would suggest a differential expression of PR isoforms in the two main cell types of the endometrium, and opens a new field of research for PR-specific molecules. Such differential expression patterns in the endometrial compartment combined with the relative proportional expression of the two receptor isoforms in the same cell type suggests that these receptors play an important role in the expression of specific genes in response to sex steroid hormones.

Mechanism of ER and PR action

On entering a target cell estrogens and progestogens interact with their respective receptors (Figure 4.4). In the classical scenario, chaperone proteins (heat-shock proteins) hold the receptors in an inactive state that changes when ligand binds. Although there is no direct evidence to suggest what happens to the receptor when ligand binds, it is thought that a conformational change occurs in the receptor and the heat-shock proteins are released and recycled[78]. The receptors in their new conformational state dimerize and then translocate to the nucleus, or translocate to the nucleus and then form a dimer that can then interact with DNA to alter transcription[79,80]. At present it is not proven which event occurs first, but the consensus is that dimerization occurs prior to nuclear translocation. The outcome, however, is that receptor dimer appears in the nucleus, where it directly contacts and interacts with palindromic sequences called hormone response elements (HREs) specific for that hormone. Thus, the hormone response element for estrogen is called the estrogen response element (ERE) and the response element for the progesterone receptor is called the progesterone response element (PRE)[81].

These elements are usually found upstream of the transcriptional start site of target genes (for simple explanations of transcriptional regulation see reference 82), in either the promoter or the enhancer region. EREs and PREs can also be found in the open-reading frame and first exons and introns[83]. Once bound to the target HRE, the receptor dimer acts as a transcriptional regulator to modulate the synthesis of specific mRNAs and proteins, thereby transmitting the effect of the specific steroid to the target cell[83]. However, often the ERE or PRE is located several hundred or thousand base pairs away from the transcriptional start site. Recent research has uncovered how ligand-bound receptors influence transcription when they are so far away from the transcriptional start site, which has also led to a better understanding of steroid hormone action (see references 76, 84 and 85 for an in-depth discussion).

The above general mechanism of action of steroid hormone receptors holds true for many situations, but cannot explain all the observations that come from the clinic and provide new challenges in the laboratory. For example, the use of anti-estrogens (such as tamoxifen) in the treatment of estrogen-dependent breast cancer causes a significant inhibition in the progression of breast cancer for the majority of patients[86]. However, tamoxifen also causes a marked increase in endometrial pathologies directly linked to the drug[86]. This discovery of the dual activities of tamoxifen created a new term for synthetic estrogens, 'selective estrogen receptor modulators (SERMs)', since tamoxifen (and many others synthesized since) have receptor agonist activities in one tissue and antagonist activities in another. However, many of the terms used to describe estrogen receptor activation and function were derived at a time when only one functional receptor was known. The recent discovery of an alternative ER, ERβ, adds another level of complexity to our understanding. The discovery of ERβ has also given important clues to the mechanism of estrogenic and anti-estrogenic action in the postmenopausal woman in the breast, brain, vasculature, bone and endometrium[27].

Receptor dimerization

The discovery of multiple ER and PR isoforms has opened the possibility that the liganded receptors can form both homodimers and heterodimers with each other to modulate gene expression[87,88]. In the classical scenario (Figure 4.5) the receptor forms a homodimer which binds to the HRE to alter transcription[87]. Recent *in vitro* data suggest that ERα and ERβ homodimers will form on consensus EREs and natural EREs[89,90]. There is also increasing evidence that an ERα–ERβ heterodimer

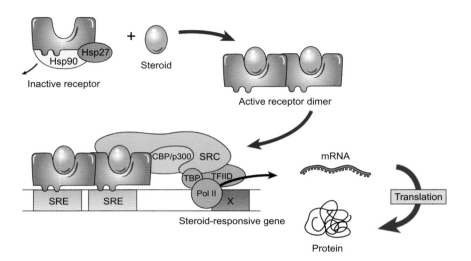

Figure 4.4. Generalized steroid hormone action via the steroid receptor. In a cell that responds to exogenous steroid hormone, the cognitive steroid receptor is held in an inactive state by chaperone proteins such as heat-shock proteins 27 (Hsp27) or 90 (Hsp90). On binding steroid hormone, the receptor undergoes a conformational change to become activated and dimerizes. On entering the nucleus the dimerized receptor hormone complex binds to chromatin sequences specific for that steroid receptor (steroid response element (SRE)), usually a palindrome of a hexamer base sequence separated by 1, 3, 4 or 5 base pairs. The next step is the recruitment of CREB-binding protein family members (CBP) and p160 family members (steroid receptor co-activators (SRC)) that interact with the dimerized steroid receptors and proteins of the basal transcriptional machinery: TATA binding protein (TBP); transcription factor IID (TFIID); and RNA polymerase II (Pol II) to increase basal transcription of the steroid-responsive gene X. This leads to increased mRNA and, via translation of the mRNA, increased protein for the X gene

will also form on natural and synthetic EREs to modulate reporter plasmid activities[88,91]. The natural extension of that theory is that cells that contain both ERα and ERβ proteins can create three possible transactivating factor combinations – ERα homodimers, ERβ homodimers and ERα–ERβ heterodimers. This has subsequently been shown to be true for several experimental systems[88,91]. However, there is another possibility that is known to occur for other family members, such as the thyroid hormone receptors and retinoic X receptor (RXR), where a single activated receptor binds to a so-called HRE half-site[92]. In most cases the half-sites perform as repressors of transcription and so are generally known as negative

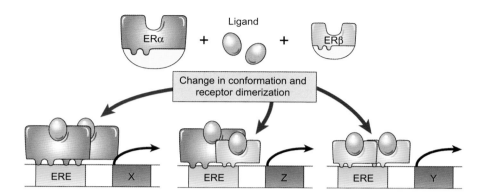

Figure 4.5. Estrogen receptors ERα and ERβ can form homodimers and heterodimers. In cell types that express both ER isoforms, such as the breast, ovary and endometrial epithelium, the same activation mechanism for the two ERs occurs as for the general steroid hormone receptor described in Figure 4.4. The same conformational change revealing the dimerization domains and the DNA binding domains occurs, allowing the receptors to form dimers and to bind to their specific steroid response elements, called estrogen response elements (EREs). In general the ERE is the palindrome sequence AGGTCA separated by three nucleotide bases, although other sequences can also act as EREs. When dimers are formed on EREs in cells that express both receptors, the dimer can form either as an ERα homodimer, an ERβ homodimer, or as an ERα–ERβ heterodimer. Cell types that contain only ERα protein (such as hepatocytes) can only form ERα homodimers and cells that express only ERβ protein (such as ovarian granulosa cells, or prostate epithelia) can only form ERβ homodimers. This raises the possibility of competition between promoter regions of several genes for receptor dimers, with the transcription of hypothetical genes X and Z affected by depletion of ERα protein and genes Y and Z affected by depletion of ERβ protein. Therefore differential gene expression in a cell that expresses both ERs will be a balance between ER expression rates and promoter requirements

response elements[93]. The agonist-activated ERα is known to bind as a single entity to the half-site ERE, but in this case acts as an activator of transcription[94], acting as a 'promiscuous partner' with the AP-1 complex to activate transcription. This raises yet another possibility – that sex steroid hormones can modulate gene transcription via heterodimerization with non-steroid hormone receptor proteins in cells that express all the component proteins.

The liganded progesterone receptor binds to the PRE as a dimer and so has the ability to bind as a PR_A homodimer, PR_B homodimer or a PR_A–PR_B heterodimer[81]. But, unlike the ER isoforms, the PRs appear to be 'faithful' and do not heterodimerize with non-steroid proteins when binding to their PRE. However, a recent report of endometrial adenocarcinoma suggests that the PR can interact with AP-1 proteins to modulate transcription, similarly to the ER–AP-1 interaction[95]. Nevertheless, it is unlikely that PRs bind to half-site PREs in the same manner that ERα does, although this has not been tested extensively, and should not be ruled out for some tissues. For example, some progestogens have androgenic-like effects in some tissues, suggesting that they can bind to the androgen receptor (AR) and androgens can bind to the PRs[96]. It has been shown that this occurs *in vitro* and that ligands will cross-react with each other's receptors, but they do not appear to transactivate genes in reporter assays[97,98]. Conversely, the recent discovery of a second AR[99,100] suggests that we should rethink how these receptors are involved in the regulation of genes in the endometrium, since androgen interferes with progesterone action and ARs are expressed in the endometrium[101,102]. 'Cross-talk' between the ERs, PRs and ARs to modulate uterine-specific gene expression is thus a real possibility[31].

As stated earlier, the HREs are often found at great distances from the transcriptional start site, and intense research into how these molecules interact with the general transcriptional machinery has identified some 'key players' in sex steroid hormone action and the mechanisms involved.

CO-REGULATORS

One of the most significant advances in recent years in the study of steroid hormone receptor action has been the discovery of steroid receptor co-regulators[103]. There are two classes of co-regulator, the co-activators and the co-repressors, and expression of both is required for efficient transcriptional regulation by nuclear receptors[104,105]. Nuclear receptor co-activators are nuclear proteins that interact with steroid receptor proteins to enhance their transcriptional activity, whereas co-repressors are proteins that interact to inhibit steroid receptor transcriptional activity. *In vitro* experiments have shown that the co-activators are the rate-limiting step for receptor activation and act as bridging proteins between the dimerized receptor and proteins of the basal transcriptional machinery (Figure 4.4)[106]. The co-repressors at present appear to be confined to the so-called type II receptor subfamily receptors (such as thyroid hormone, retinoic X, retinoic acid, vitamin D and peroxisome proliferator-activated receptors), although several hypotheses have been proposed that suggest that for certain cell types ERα and co-repressors bind to cause antagonistic activity, which can be overcome by a stronger ligand, whereas co-activators bind to enhance gene transcription[107]. In contrast there are several co-activator proteins that activate both type I (ER, PR, AR, mineralocorticoid receptors and glucocorticoid receptors (GR)) and some type II receptors.

The main group of co-activator proteins belongs to the steroid receptor co-activator (SRC) family (now termed the p160 family of co-activators), of which the SRC-1 protein is the prototypical factor. SRC-1 was the first member of this family of proteins that dramatically enhances the transcriptional activity of steroid receptors to be cloned[108]. The SRC proteins physically interact with ERα, ERβ and PR in a ligand-dependent manner[78,109] to increase their transcriptional activity through interaction with α-helix 12, which is part of the receptor's LBD[27]. Experiments have shown that SRC proteins are essential for efficient transmission of sex steroid hormone signaling on gene transcription. Direct injection of anti-SRC-1 antibodies into cells inhibits steroid-dependent transcription, indicating that these molecules are essential for efficient transcription and are rate limiting[110]. Other elegant experiments have shown that over-expression of SRC-1 can overcome the squelching effect of ERα on progesterone-dependent transcription, suggesting that SRC-1 interferes with the interaction between ERα and PR-dependent signaling pathways[108]. Although SRC-1 binds directly to both ER isoforms and both PR isoforms, it also maintains the ability to alter the conformation of adjacent chromatin. This is the main function of SRC-1 and other p160 family members, to bridge the sex hormone receptor–response element complex basal transcriptional machinery and to open chromatin to make transcription occur more efficiently. SRC-1 has intrinsic histone acetyltransferase (HAT) activity, similar to that of the natural nuclear histone acetyltransferases[111], which are key enzymes that control the unwinding of DNA from the condensed histone–DNA complexes, making the DNA more accessible to the transcriptional machinery (Figure 4.6). The other members of the SRC family – called SRC-2 and SRC-3 – also enhance the transcriptional activities of several nuclear receptors, including ERα and PR_A[112–114], but not ERβ or PR_B, suggesting that other proteins or mechanisms are required for these two receptor proteins. This may be true, because one recent report has indicated that SRC-3 (also known as AIB1 or TRAM-1) selectively enhances ERα transcription over that of ERβ, presumably because of subtle sequence differences in the LBD of these two receptors[115].

The list of steroid receptor co-activators is increasing daily and no doubt more will be found, but of the large number that are already recognized two require special mention here. The first is cAMP response element binding activity (CREB)-binding protein (CBP). CBP is a general co-activator for many nuclear transcription factors including p53, STAT-2 and of course CREB[116]. However CBP also enhances ERα and PR transcription *in vitro*[104,110,117]. CBP also interacts with SRC-1 and with the

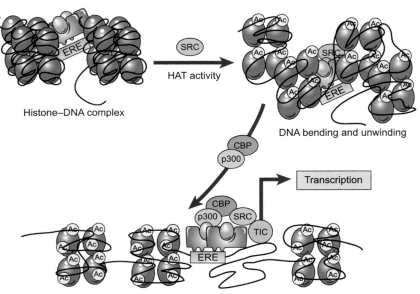

Histone–DNA complex

HAT activity

SRC

DNA bending and unwinding

CBP
p300

Transcription

CBP
p300 SRC
TIC

ERE

Estrogen-responsive gene efficiently transcribed

Figure 4.6. The role of steroid receptor co-activator (SRC) in enhancing estrogen-dependent transcription. The DNA of an estrogen-responsive gene is normally tightly regulated with respect to its basal transcription. The histone–DNA complex consists of multimeric histone proteins with DNA wound tightly around it. The estrogen response element (ERE) of a target is available for binding of dimerized estrogen receptor (ER) proteins and recruitment of SRC proteins. The SRC proteins and related p160 co-activators have intrinsic histone acetyltransferase (HAT) activity, that acetylates key terminal amino groups of lysine residues (yellow circles) on the histone H2A, H2B, H3 and H4 proteins, causing the histone–DNA complex to destabilize and a general bending or unwinding of the DNA sequence. This allows the recruitment of accessory factors such as the CREB-binding protein (CBP)/p300 and other co-integrators (shown as red and pink circles) that enhance the acetylation process further to completely unwind the DNA from the histone proteins. This opens the entire reading frame of the target gene and allows more efficient interaction between the steroid hormone receptor, SRC, CBP and proteins of the transcription initiation complex (TIC) so that enhanced transcription occurs, leading to increased levels of transcript

steroid receptor in a synergistic manner, suggesting that CBP could act as a mediator of different signaling pathways that converge at a single point, the transactivation of the steroid-inducible gene. Indeed, other evidence tends to support this idea. An adenovirus E1A-associated 300-kDa protein (p300), very similar in its structure to SRC family members, acts as a co-activator for other nuclear transcription factors, such as nuclear factor-κB (NF-κB) and the tumor-suppressor protein p53[104].

A second steroid receptor co-activator that needs to be mentioned is the steroid receptor RNA activator (SRA), because it is unusual in several respects. SRA selectively enhances the activity of PR, ER, GR and AR but not other nuclear receptors such as thyroid hormone receptors and RXR[118]. Moreover, SRA acts to increase gene transcription as an RNA transcript and not as a protein, yet it still interacts with steroid receptors to enhance their activity. The proof that SRA acts as an RNA molecule rather than as a protein is shown by its ability to enhance transcription in the presence of cycloheximide (an inhibitor of protein translation), whereas SRC-1 cannot[118]. This indicates that SRC-1 action requires the production of nascent protein, whereas SRA action does not. In addition SRA appears to function through interaction with AF-1 of the ERα, whereas most co-activators and co-repressors interact with AF-2 in the LBD of steroid receptors (Figure 4.7). However, recent evidence suggests that ligand-independent phosphorylation of ERβ causes the recruitment of SRC-1 to the AF-1 region of ERβ, whereas estradiol binding to ERβ causes recruitment of SRC-1 to the AF-2 region. This suggests that cells that express different co-activators and co-repressors have much better control over steroid receptor transcription than cells that express a different repertoire of co-regulators. Interestingly, the expression of a 203-bp variant of SRA appears to be linked to an increased risk for breast cancer[119]. These data suggest that more complex mechanisms may be involved in the regulation of steroid hormone action than is known at present.

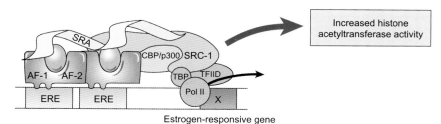

Estrogen-responsive gene

Figure 4.7. The effect of co-activators on estrogen receptor (ERα) gene transactivation. p160 co-activators such as steroid receptor co-activator-1 (SRC-1) bind to the dimerized ER–estrogen response element (ERE) complex via the ligand-dependent transcription activation function AF-2. With further recruitment of other proteins such as CREB-binding protein (CBP)/p300, increased histone acetyltransferase activity occurs to unwind the histone–DNA complex, as outlined in Figure 4.6. The steroid receptor RNA activator (SRA) co-activator is an RNA molecule that interacts with the transcription activator function AF-1 in either the absence or presence of CBP/p300 and SRC-1 to activate histone acetyltransferase. At present it is not known if both mechanisms are mutually exclusive or work together to enhance gene transcription, but SRA may interact with p160 co-activators. The net outcome of both co-activator binders is increased histone acetyltransferase activity. Pol II, RNA polymerase II; TBP, TATA binding protein; TFIID, transcription factor IID

CONCLUSION

This review has highlighted some of the newer advances made in recent years to aid – and complicate – our understanding of the molecular mechanisms behind steroid hormone action. A global understanding of gene regulation by nuclear receptors, including the ERs and PRs, will provide us with knowledge that can be used to devise better treatments for conditions that affect the postmenopausal woman, including some gynecologic disorders, osteoporosis, atherosclerosis and senile dementia.

REFERENCES

1. Greendale GA, Lee NP, Arriola ER. The menopause. *Lancet* 1999;353:571–80
2. Sherwin BB. Hormones, mood, and cognitive functioning in postmenopausal women. *Obstet Gynecol* 1996;87(Suppl 2):20S–26S
3. Sherwin BB. Can estrogen keep you smart? Evidence from clinical studies. *J Psychiatry Neurosci* 1999;24:315–21
4. Lindsay R. The role of estrogen in the prevention of osteoporosis. *Endocrinol Metab Clin North Am* 1998;27:399–409
5. The ESHRE Capri Workshop Group. Hormones and cardiovascular diseases: oral contraceptives and hormonal replacement therapy: differential effects on coronary heart disease, deep venous thrombosis and stroke. *Hum Reprod* 1998;13:2325–33
6. Kanis JA. Estrogens, the menopause, and osteoporosis. *Bone* 1996;19:185S–190S
7. Suh Y-H, Chong YH, Kim S-H, *et al*. Molecular physiology, biochemistry, and pharmacology of Alzheimer's amyloid precursor protein (APP). *Ann N Y Acad Sci* 1996;786:169–83
8. Brandi ML, Becherini L, Gennari L, *et al*. Association of the estrogen receptor α gene polymorphisms with sporadic Alzheimer's disease. *Biochem Biophys Res Commun* 1999; 265:335–8
9. Huezo CM. Current reversible contraceptive methods: a global perspective. *Int J Gynaecol Obstet* 1998;62(Suppl 1):S3–S15
10. Christin-Maitre S, Bouchard P, Spitz IM. Medical termination of pregnancy. *N Engl J Med* 2000;342:946–56
11. Spitz IM, Croxatto HB, Robbins A. Antiprogestins: mechanism of action and contraceptive potential. *Annu Rev Pharmacol Toxicol* 1996;36:47–81
12. Fisher B, Powles TJ, Pritchard KJ. Tamoxifen for the prevention of breast cancer. *Eur J Cancer* 2000;36:142–50
13. MacGregor JI, Jordan VC. Basic guide to the mechanism of antiestrogen action. *Endocr Rev* 1998;50:151–96
14. Levy D, Christin-Maitre S, Leroy I, *et al*. The endometrial approach in contraception. *Ann N Y Acad Sci* 1997;828:59–83

15. Loret de Mola JR. Endometrial changes with chronic tamoxifen use. *Curr Opin Obstet Gynecol* 1997;9:160–4

16. Beato M, Klug J. Steroid receptors: an update. *Hum Reprod Update* 2000;6:225–36

17. Fuller PJ. The steroid receptor superfamily: mechanisms of diversity. *FASEB J* 1991;5:3092–9

18. Inoue S, Hashino S-J, Miyoshi H, *et al*. Identification of a novel isoform of estrogen receptor, a potential inhibitor of estrogen action, in vascular smooth muscle cells. *Biochem Biophys Res Commun* 1996;219:766–72

19. Weigel NL. Steroid hormone receptors and their regulation by phosphorylation. *Biochem J* 1996;319:657–67

20. Beato M, Herrlich P, Schutz G. Steroid hormone receptors: many actors in search of a plot. *Cell* 1995;83:851–7

21. Moras D, Gronemeyer H. The nuclear receptor ligand-binding domain: structure and function. *Curr Opin Cell Biol* 1998;10:384–91

22. Gronemeyer H. Transcription activation by nuclear receptors. *J Receptor Res* 1993;13:667–91

23. Mueller-Fahrnow A, Egner U. Ligand-binding domain of estrogen receptors. *Curr Opin Biotechnol* 1999;10:550–6

24. Greene GL, Gilna P, Waterfield M, *et al*. Sequence and expression of human estrogen receptor complementary DNA. *Science* 1986;231:1150–4

25. Kuiper GGJM, Enmark E, Pelto-Huikko M, *et al*. Cloning of a novel estrogen receptor expressed in rat prostate and ovary. *Proc Natl Acad Sci USA* 1996;93:5925–30

26. Mosselman S, Polman J, Dijkema R, *et al*. ER beta: identification and characterization of a novel estrogen receptor. *FEBS Lett* 1996;392:49–53

27. Muramatsu M, Inoue S. Estrogen receptors: how do they control reproductive and nonreproductive functions? *Biochem Biophys Res Commun* 2000;270:1–10

28. Sun J, Meyers MJ, Fink BE, *et al*. Novel ligands that function as selective estrogens or antiestrogens for estrogen receptor-alpha or estrogen receptor-beta. *Endocrinology* 1999;140:800–4

29. Enmark E, Gustafsson JA. Oestrogen receptors – an overview. *J Intern Med* 1999;246:133–8

30. Paech K, Webb P, Kuiper GG, *et al*. Differential ligand activation of estrogen receptors ERalpha and ERbeta at AP1 sites. *Science* 1997;277:1508–10

31. Katzenellenbogen BS. Mechanisms of action and cross-talk between estrogen receptor and progesterone receptor pathways. *J Soc Gynecol Invest* 2000;7(Suppl 1):S33–7

32. McDonnell DP. The molecular pharmacology of SERMs. *Trends Endocrinol Metab* 1999;10:301–11

33. Cano A, Hermenegildo C. The endometrial effects of SERMs. *Hum Reprod Update* 2000;6:244–54

34. Taylor JA, Lewis KJ, Lubajn DB. Estrogen receptor mutations. *Mol Cell Endocrinol* 1998;145:61–6

35. Ma CH, Dong KW, Yu KL. cDNA cloning and expression of a novel estrogen receptor beta-subtype in goldfish (*Carassius auratus*). *Biochim Biophys Acta* 2000;1490:145–52

36. Asaithambi A, Mukherjee S, Thakur MK. Expression of 112-kDa estrogen receptor in mouse brain cortex and its autoregulation with age. *Biochem Biophys Res Commun* 1997;231:683–5

37. Ikeuchi T, Todo T, Koyabashi T, *et al.* cDNA cloning of a novel androgen receptor subtype. *J Biol Chem* 1999;274:25205–9

38. Chiadarun SS, Alexander JM. A tumor-specific truncated estrogen receptor splice variant enhances estrogen-stimulated gene expression. *Mol Endocrinol* 1998;12:1355–66

39. Resnick EM, Schreihofer DA, Periasamy A, *et al.* Truncated estrogen receptor product-1 suppresses estrogen receptor transactivation by dimerization with estrogen receptors alpha and beta. *J Biol Chem* 2000;275:7158–66

40. Rice LW, Jazaeri AA, Shupnik MA. Estrogen receptor mRNA splice variants in pre- and postmenopausal human endometrium and endometrial carcinoma. *Gynecol Oncol* 1997;65:149–57

41. Jones PS, Parrott E, White INH. Activation of transcription by estrogen receptor alpha and beta is cell type- and promoter-dependent. *J Biol Chem* 1999;274:32008–14

42. Wakeling AE. Similarities and distinctions in the mode of action of different classes of antioestrogens. *Endocr Relat Cancer* 2000;7:17–28

43. Webb P, Nguyen P, Valentine C, *et al.* The estrogen receptor enhances AP-1 activity by two distinct mechanisms with different requirements for receptor transactivation functions. *Mol Endocrinol* 1999;13:1672–85

44. Fujimoto J, Hirose R, Ichigo S, *et al.* Expression of progesterone receptor form A and B mRNAs in uterine leiomyomata. *Tumour Biol* 1998;19:126–31

45. Tora L, Gronemeyer H, Turcotte B, *et al.* The N-terminal region of the chicken progesterone receptor specifies target gene activation. *Nature (London)* 1988;333:185–8

46. Chalbos D, Galtier F. Differential effect of forms A and B of human progesterone receptor on estradiol-dependent transcription. *J Biol Chem* 1994;269:23007–12

47. Wang H, Critchley HOD, Kelly RW, *et al.* Progesterone receptor subtype B is differentially regulated in human endometrial stroma. *Mol Hum Reprod* 1998;4:407–12

48. Noe M, Kunz G, Herbertz M, *et al.* The cyclic pattern of the immunocytochemical expression of oestrogen and progesterone receptors in human myometrial and endometrial layers: characterization of the endometrial-subendometrial unit. *Hum Reprod* 1999;14:190–7

49. Moutsatsou P, Sekeris CE. Estrogen and progesterone receptors in the endometrium. *Ann N Y Acad Sci* 1997;816:99–115

50. Camacho-Arroyo I, Pasapera AM, Cerbon MA. Regulation of progesterone receptor gene expression by sex steroid hormones in the hypothalamus and the cerebral cortex of the rabbit. *Neurosci Lett* 1996;214:25–8

51. Macpherson AM, Archer DF, Leslie S, *et al.* The effect of estronogestrel on VEGF, oestrogen and progesterone receptor immunoreactivity and endothelial cell number in human endometrium. *Hum Reprod* 1999;14:3080–7

52. Iafrati MD, Karas RH, Aronovitz M, *et al.* Estrogen inhibits the vascular injury response in estrogen receptor alpha-deficient mice. *Nature Med* 1997;3:545–8

53. Lauber AH, Romano GJ, Pfaff DW. Gene expression for estrogen and progesterone receptor mRNAs in rat brain and possible relations to sexually dimorphic functions. *J Steroid Biochem Mol Biol* 1991;40:53–62

54. Onoe Y, Miyaura C, Ohta H, *et al.* Expression of estrogen receptor beta in rat bone. *Endocrinology* 1997;138:4509–12

55. Shughrue PJ, Komm B, Merchentaler I. The distribution of estrogen receptor-beta mRNA in the rat hypothalamus. *Steroids* 1996;61:678–81

56. Graham JD, Clarke CL. Physiological action of progesterone in target tissues. *Endocr Rev* 1997;18:502–19

57. McEwen BS. Clinical review 108: The molecular and neuroanatomical basis for estrogen effects in the central nervous system. *J Clin Endocrinol Metab* 1999;84:1790–7

58. Hodson J, Thompson J, Al-Azzawi F. Headache at menopause and in hormone replacement therapy users. *Climacteric* 2000;3:119–24

59. Steiner H, Haass C. Intramembrane proteolysis by presenilins. *Nat Rev Mol Cell Biol* 2000;1:217–24

60. Mattila KM, Axelman K, Rinne JO, *et al.* Interaction between estrogen receptor 1 and the epsilon4 allele of apolipoprotein E increases the risk of familial Alzheimer's disease in women. *Neurosci Lett* 2000;282:45–8

61. Healy DL, Hodgen GD. The endocrinology of human endometrium. *Obstet Gynecol Surv* 1983;38:509–30

62. Snijders M, DeGoeij A, Debets-Te Baerts MJC, *et al.* Immunocytochemical analysis of oestrogen receptors and progesterone receptors in the human uterus throughout the menstrual cycle and after the menopause. *J Reprod Fertil* 1992;94:363–71

63. Tseng L, Zhu HH. Regulation of progesterone receptor messenger ribonucleic acid by progestin in human endometrial stromal cells. *Biol Reprod* 1997;57:1360–6

64. Fujishita A, Nakane PK, Koji T, *et al.* Expression of estrogen and progesterone receptors in endometrium and peritoneal endometriosis: an immunohistochemical and *in situ* hybridization study. *Fertil Steril* 1997;67:856–64

65. Matsuzaki S, Fukaya T, Suzuki T, *et al.* Oestrogen receptor alpha and beta mRNA expression in human endometrium throughout the menstrual cycle. *Mol Hum Reprod* 1999;5:559–64

66. Saville B, Wormke M, Wang F, *et al.* Ligand-, cell-, and estrogen receptor subtype (alpha/beta)-dependent activation at GC-rich (Sp1) promoter elements. *J Biol Chem* 2000;275:5379–87

67. Zou K, Ing NH. Oestradiol up-regulates oestrogen receptor, cyclophilin, and glyceraldehyde phosphate dehydrogenase mRNA concentrations in endometrium, but down-regulates them in the liver. *J Steroid Biochem Mol Biol* 1998;46:231–7

68. Santagati S, Gianazza E, Agrati P, *et al.* Oligonucleotide squelching reveals the mechanism of estrogen receptor autologous down-regulation. *Mol Endocrinol* 1997;11:938–49

69. Kastner P, Krust A, Turcotte B, *et al.* Two distinct estrogen-regulated promoters generate transcripts encoding the two functionally different human progesterone receptor forms A and B. *EMBO J* 1990;9:1603–14

70. Savouret JF, Rauch M, Redeuilh G, *et al.* Interplay between estrogens, progestins, retinoic acid and AP-1 on a single regulatory site in the progesterone receptor gene. *J Biol Chem* 1994;269:28955–62

71. Leavitt WW, Toft DO, Strott CA, *et al.* Specific progesterone receptor in the hamster uterus: physiologic properties and regulation during the estrous cycle. *Endocrinology* 1974;94:1041–53

72. Kreitmann B, Bugat R, Bayard F. Estrogen and progestin regulation of the progesterone receptor concentration in human endometrium. *J Clin Endocrinol Metab* 1979;49:926–9

73. Couse JF, Korach KS. Estrogen receptor null mice: what have we learned and where will they lead us? *Endocr Rev* 1999;20:358–417

74. Tibbetts TA, Conneely OM, O'Malley BW. Progesterone via its receptor antagonizes the pro-inflammatory activity of estrogen in the mouse uterus. *Biol Reprod* 1999;60:1158–65

75. Conneely OM, Lydon JP, De Mayo F, *et al.* Reproductive functions of the progesterone receptor. *J Soc Gynecol Invest* 2000;7(Suppl 1):S25–32

76. Vegeto E, Wagner BL, Imhof MO, *et al.* The molecular pharmacology of ovarian steroid receptors. *Vitam Horm* 1996;52:99–128

77. Vegeto E, Shahbaz MM, Wen DX, *et al.* Human progesterone receptor A form is a cell- and promoter-specific repressor of human progesterone receptor B function. *Mol Endocrinol* 1993;7:1244–55

78. Kraichely DM, Sun J, Katzenellenbogen JA, *et al.* Conformational changes and coactivator recruitment by novel ligands for estrogen receptor-α and esrogen receptor-β: correlations with biological character and distinct differences among SRC coactivator family members. *Endocrinology* 2000;141:3534–45

79. Brinkmann AO. Steroid hormone receptors: activators of gene transcription. *J Pediatr Endocrinol* 1994;7:275–82

80. Smith CO, O'Malley BW. Evolving concepts of selective estrogen receptor action: from basic science to clinical applications. *Trends Endocrinol Metab* 1999;10:299–300

81. Leonhardt SA, Altmann M, Edwards DP. Agonists and antagonists induce homo-dimerization and mixed ligand heterodimerization of human progesterone receptors *in vivo* by a mammalian two-hybrid assay. *Mol Endocrinol* 1998;12:1914–30

82. Taylor AH. Fundamental gene expression. *CME Bull Gynaecol* 1998;1:25

83. McDonnell DP, Clevenger B, Dana S, *et al.* The mechanism of action of steroid hormones: a new twist to an old tale. *J Clin Pharmacol* 1993;33:1165–72

84. Brann DW, Hendry LB, Mahesh VB. Emerging diversities in the mechanism of action of steroid hormones. *J Steroid Biochem Mol Biol* 1995;52:113–33

85. Williams GR, Franklyn JA. Physiology of the steroid-thyroid hormone nuclear receptor superfamily. *Baillière's Clin Endocrinol Metab* 1994;8:241–66

86. Jordan VC, Morrow M. Tamoxifen, raloxifene, and the prevention of breast cancer. *Endocr Rev* 1999;20:253–78

87. Truss M, Beato M. Steroid hormone receptors: interaction with deoxyribonucleic acid and transcription factors. *Endocr Rev* 1993;14:459–79

88. Pace P, Taylor J, Suntharalingam S, *et al.* Human estrogen receptor beta binds DNA in a manner similar to and dimerizes with estrogen receptor alpha. *J Biol Chem* 1997;272: 25832–8

89. Brandt ME, Vickery LE. Cooperativity and dimerization of recombinant human estrogen receptor hormone-binding domain. *J Biol Chem* 1997;272:4843–9

90. Cowley SM, Hoare S, Mosselman S, *et al.* Estrogen receptors alpha and beta form heterodimers on DNA. *J Biol Chem* 1997;272:19858–62

91. Pettersson K, Grandien K, Kuiper G, *et al.* Mouse estrogen receptor beta forms estrogen response element-binding heterodimers with estrogen receptor alpha. *Mol Endocrinol* 1997;11:1486–96

92. Sheppard MC, Franklyn JA, Yarwood NJ, *et al.* Thyroid hormone regulation of human pituitary alpha subunit gene expression. *Acta Med Austriaca* 1992;19(Suppl 1):66–8

93. Taylor AH, Wishart P, Lawless DE, *et al*. Identification of functional positive and negative thyroid hormone-responsive elements in the rat apolipoprotein AI promoter. *Biochemistry* 1996;35:8281–8

94. Crowe DL, Brown TN, Kim R, *et al*. A c-*fos*/estrogen receptor fusion protein promotes cell cycle progression and proliferation of human cancer cell lines. *Mol Cell Biol Res Commun* 2000;3:243–8

95. Bamberger AM, Bamberger CM, Gellersen B, *et al*. Modulation of AP-1 activity by the human progesterone receptor in endometrial adenocarcinoma cells. *Proc Natl Acad Sci USA* 1996;93:6169–74

96. Bergink EW, van Meel F, Turpijn EW, *et al*. Binding of progestagens to receptor proteins in MCF-7 cells. *J Steroid Biochem* 1983;19:1563–70

97. Janne OA, Bardin CW. Steroid receptors and hormone action: physiological and synthetic androgens and progestins can mediate inappropriate biological effects. *Pharmacol Rev* 1984;36(Suppl 2):35S–42S

98. Grody WW, Schrader WT, O'Malley BW. Activation, transformation, and subunit structure of steroid hormone receptors. *Endocr Rev* 1982;3:141–63

99. Wilson CM, McPhaul MJ. A and B forms of the androgen receptor are expressed in a variety of human tissues. *Mol Cell Endocrinol* 1996;120:51–7

100. Gao T, McPhaul MJ. Functional activities of the A and B forms of the human androgen receptor in response to androgen receptor agonists and antagonists. *Mol Endocrinol* 1998;12:654–63

101. Fujimoto J, Nishigaki M, Hori M, *et al*. Biological implications of estrogen and androgen effects on androgen receptor and its mRNA levels in human uterine endometrium. *Gynecol Endocrinol* 1995;9:149–55

102. Mertens HJ, Heineman MJ, Koudstaal J, *et al*. Androgen receptor content in human endometrium. *Eur J Obstet Gynecol Reprod Biol* 1996;70:11–13

103. Torchia J, Glass C, Rosenfeld MG. Co-activators and co-repressors in the integration of transcriptional responses. *Curr Opin Cell Biol* 1998;10:373–83

104. McKenna NJ, Lanz RB, O'Malley BW. Nuclear receptor coregulators: cellular and molecular biology. *Endocr Rev* 1999;20:321–44

105. Glass CK, Rosenfeld MG. The coregulator exchange in transcriptional functions of nuclear receptors. *Genes Dev* 2000;14:121–41

106. Freedman LP. Multimeric coactivator complexes for steroid/nuclear receptors. *Trends Endocrinol Metab* 1999;10:403–7

107. Onate SA, Boonyaratanakornkit V, Spencer TE, *et al*. The steroid receptor coactivator-1 contains multiple receptor interacting and activation domains that cooperatively enhance the activation function 1 (AF1) and AF2 domains of steroid receptors. *J Biol Chem* 1998;273:12101–8

108. Onate SA, Tsai SY, Tsai MJ, *et al*. Sequence and characterization of a coactivator for the steroid hormone receptor superfamily. *Science* 1995;270:1354–7

109. Clemens JW, Robker RL, Kraus WL, *et al*. Hormone induction of progesterone receptor (PR) messenger ribonucleic acid and activation of PR promoter regions in ovarian granulosa cells: evidence for a role of cyclic adenosine 3′,5′-monophosphate but not estradiol. *Mol Endocrinol* 1998;12:1201–14

110. Torchia J, Rose DW, Inostroza J, *et al.* The transcriptional co-activator p/CIP binds CBP and mediates nuclear-receptor function. *Nature (London)* 1997;387:677–84

111. Grant PA, Berger SL, Workman JL. Identification and analysis of native nucleosomal histone acetyltransferase complexes. *Methods Mol Biol* 1999;119:311–17

112. Voegel JJ, Heine MJ, Tini M, *et al.* The coactivator TIF2 contains three nuclear receptor-binding motifs and mediates transactivation through CBP binding-dependent and -independent pathways. *EMBO J* 1998;17:507–19

113. Chen D, Huang S-M, Stallcup MR. Synergistic, p160 coactivator-dependent enhancement of estrogen receptor function by CARM1 and p300. *J Biol Chem* 2000; 275:40810–16

114. Leo C, Chen JD. The SRC family of nuclear receptor coactivators. *Gene* 2000;245: 1–11

115. Suen C-S, Berrodin TJ, Mastroeni R, *et al.* A transcriptional coactivator, steroid receptor coactivator-3, selectively augments steroid receptor transcriptional activity. *J Biol Chem* 1998;273:27645–53

116. Goodman RH, Smolik S. CBP/p300 in cell growth, transformation, and development. *Genes Dev* 2000;14:1553–77

117. Kamei Y, Xu L, Heinzel T, *et al.* A CBP integrator complex mediates transcriptional activation and AP-1 inhibition by nuclear receptors. *Cell* 1996;85:403–14

118. Lanz RB, McKenna NJ, Onate SA, *et al.* A steroid receptor coactivator, SRA, functions as an RNA and is present in an SRC-1 complex. *Cell* 1999;97:17–27

119. Leygue E, Dotzlaw H, Watson PH, *et al.* Expression of the steroid receptor RNA activator in human breast tumors. *Cancer Res* 1999;59:4190–3

5
Progestogens and the endometrium
M. Habiba

INTRODUCTION

Although formal evidence of a causal link is lacking, and no mechanism has yet been established at a molecular level, clinical studies have linked unopposed estrogen replacement therapy to an increased risk of endometrial hyperplasia and cancer[1,2]. To guard against these changes, the current practice is to add a minimum of 10 days of progestogen to every 28-day treatment cycle[3]. Current evidence suggests that this is effective in preventing both endometrial hyperplasia and malignancy[4]. Progestogen is also used in the management of many other gynecologic conditions:

(1) As a contraceptive either on its own (e.g. the minipill, depot contraception or contraceptive implants) or, more commonly, combined with estrogen in the combined pill;

(2) For endometrial preparation prior to implantation in some assisted conception techniques; and

(3) For the management of menstrual disorders, particularly when cycles are irregular.

Less common indications include the treatment of endometriosis and inoperable endometrial cancer.

Progestogens are commonly administered orally, but transdermal preparations are becoming increasingly available for use in hormone replacement therapy (HRT). Other routes of administration include depot injections, transmucosally by suppositories and locally as with the use of medicated intrauterine contraceptive devices.

Progestogens act on the estrogen-primed endometrium to inhibit cell proliferation, down-regulate estrogen and progesterone receptors (ER and PR), and to stimulate the effect of 17β-estradiol dehydrogenase, the enzyme responsible for converting 17β-estradiol into the less active metabolite estrone.

In this chapter the different progestogens used in HRT and other areas of gynecology will be reviewed, with particular reference to their endometrial effects. The terms progestogen, progestin and gestagen will be used interchangeably in reference to natural or synthetic compounds.

PROGESTOGEN PREPARATIONS

Progesterone is the only natural compound that has significant progestational activity, which it induces through binding to progesterone receptors located in the nucleus. Synthetic progestogens share with natural progesterone its affinity for the specific receptor and its ability to influence secretory transformation in the estrogen-primed endometrium. The induction of certain biologic change by a particular progestogen may be independent of its ability to induce other effects. In the body progesterone is derived from cholesterol, first by hydroxylation at C-20 and C-22, followed by cleavage of the bond between C-20 and C-22 to produce pregnenolone. The latter reaction is catalyzed by desmolase and requires reduced adenine dinucleotide phosphate (NADPH) and O_2. Progesterone is synthesized from pregnenolone in two steps: first, the 3-hydroxyl group of pregnenolone is oxidized to a 3-keto group, then the Δ^5 double bond is isomerized to a Δ^4 double bond. Progesterone hydroxylation at C-11 is the initial step in the synthesis of cortical steroids and of androgens and estrogens (Figure 5.1).

Derivation of synthetic progestogen

Synthetic progestogens are made by chemical manipulation of parent compounds. While hydroxylation of progesterone at C-17 results in loss of its progestational activity, the addition of a carboxymethyl side-chain at C-17 confers stability and restores progestogenic effect on the compounds which, thus converted, can be used parenterally as long-acting agents. The parent compound for acetylated progestogens is 17-hydroxyprogesterone acetate, and the group includes: medroxyprogesterone acetate, formed by addition of a methyl group at C-6; megestrol acetate, formed by addition of a methyl group at C-6 and formation of a double bond between C-6 and C-7; and cyproterone acetate, formed by the substitution of a chlorine atom for a hydrogen at C-6, formation of a double bond between C-6 and C-7, and

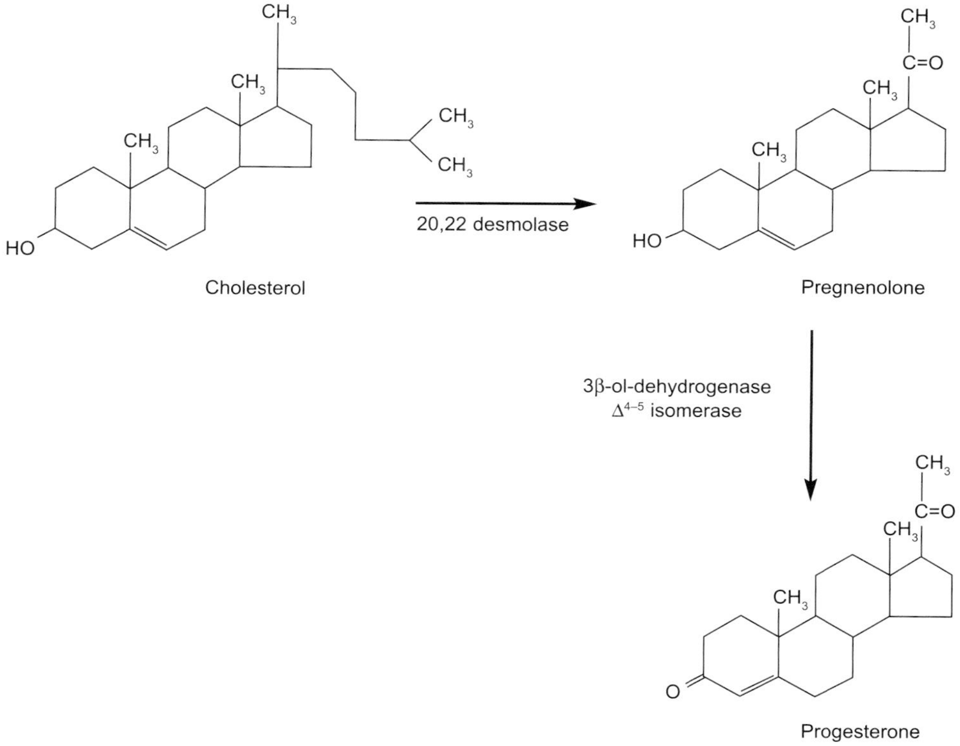

Figure 5.1. Schematic outline of the synthesis of progesterone from cholesterol

addition of a 'bridging' methylene group between C-1 and C-2 to form a three-membered ring. Other acetylated pregnane derivatives have been produced.

Progestational agents structurally related to progesterone

The only non-acetate pregnane derivative widely used is dydrogesterone, which lacks the acetate group at C-17. Its structure is similar to that of natural progesterone except for three differences: in dydrogesterone the hydrogen atom at C-9 is in the β-position, the methyl group at C-10 is in the α-position (which is the reverse arrangement to that in progesterone, hence the name 'retro' progesterone), and dydrogesterone has an additional double bond between C-6 and C-7 (Figure 5.2).

Trimegestone is a recently introduced progestogen that is structurally related to progesterone. It is a 17β[(S)-2-hydroxypropanoyl]-17-methyl-estra-4,9-dien-3-one (Figure 5.2). As is the case with the ethinylated testosterone derivative norethindrone

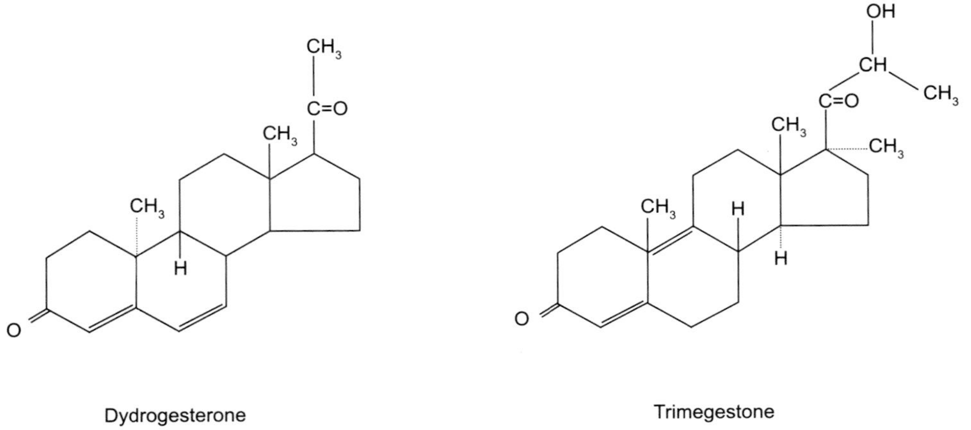

Figure 5.2. The structures of dydrogesterone and trimegestone

(see below), the angular methyl group at C-10 has been removed, which results in a further increase in potency and a reduction in androgenicity. Other members of the nor-pregnane group include demegestone and promegestone.

Progestational agents derived from ethinylated testosterone

The second group of widely used progestogens are the ethinylated testosterone derivatives. The addition of an ethinyl group at C-17 of the testosterone molecule results in loss of its androgenic potency, and in its acquisition of progestogenic properties. It also confers stability for oral use. Norethisterone (norethindrone) can be regarded as being derived from 17α-ethinyltestosterone by removal of the methyl group at C-10[5]. Other synthetic compounds known to be converted in the human body into norethisterone are lynestrenol, norethynodrel, norethisterone acetate and ethynodiol diacetate (Figure 5.3).

Norgestrel is derived from 17α-ethinyltestosterone by removal of the C-10 methyl group and the substitution of an ethyl for a methyl group at C-13. Synthesized norgestrel is a racemic mixture of an active levo form and the inactive dextro form. Levonorgestrel (LNG) itself is one of the most potent progestogens. Others include its derivatives (genane derivatives) or the 'third generation' contraceptive progestogens (norgestimate, desogestrel and gestodene). These are formed by substitutions in the steroid rings of the parent compound (Figure 5.4).

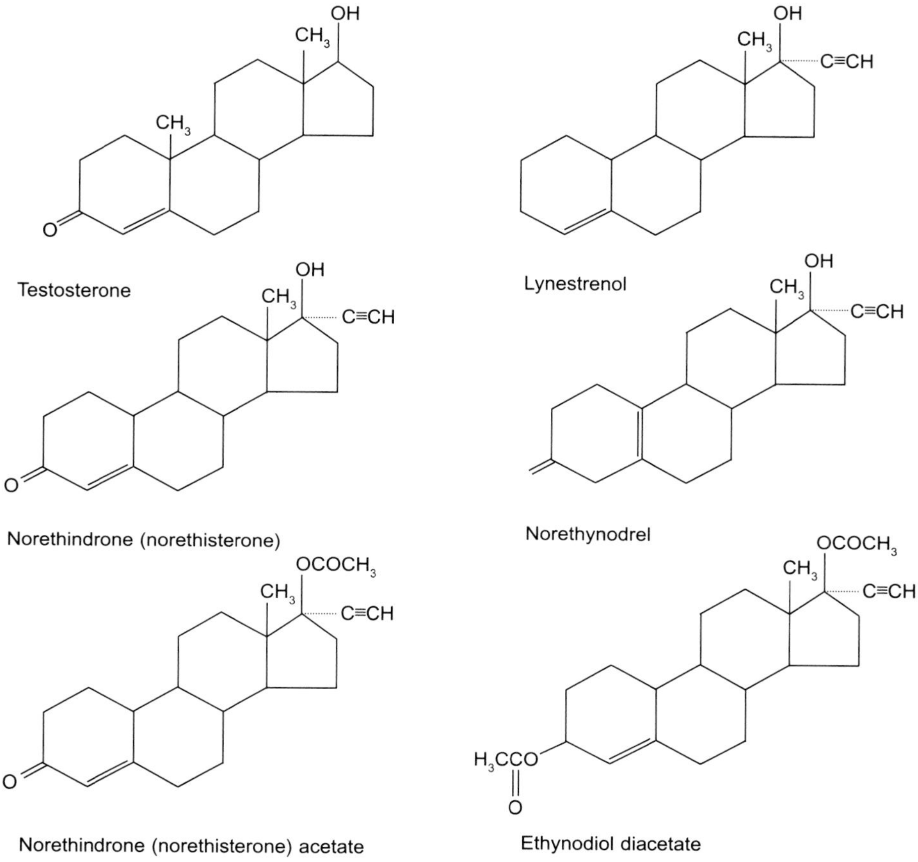

Figure 5.3. The structures of norethindrone and related progestogens compared to testosterone

A more recently introduced progestogen is nestorone, 16-methylene-17-acetoxy-19-norpregn-4-ene-3,20-dione, which has been shown to be 10–100 times more potent than progesterone when administered parenterally, but to be relatively inactive when used orally[6]. Such compounds have considerable potential as sustained release preparations. Other recent developments have been directed towards the development of progestogen antagonists such as RU486, ZK 98.299 and ZK 98.734.

Progestogenic potency

As mentioned above, progestogenic potency is dependent on receptor binding, which in turn is dependent on bioavailability, binding affinity and elimination. In

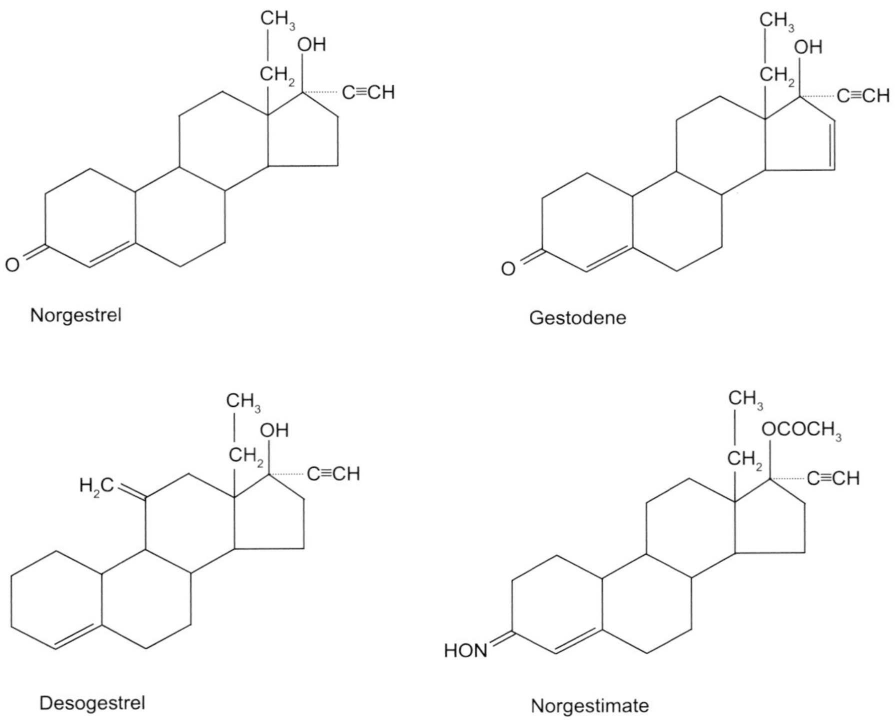

Figure 5.4. Norgestrel and third-generation progestogens

practice, progestogenic potency and estrogenic and androgenic potency are measured with reference to the parent compound, but difficulties arise in relation to the definition of the typical effect of the reference compound itself. This may be species-dependent, and may vary according to the assay used, thus a compound may be more effective in inducing one but not other effects. This is further complicated in the case of progestogens and some other steroids in two ways: firstly, these compounds are metabolized at different rates to different intermediate and end-products that may not themselves be inert. Secondly, steroids and their metabolites have different affinities for androgen and other steroid receptors, which confer on the compound properties besides those typical of their class.

It has long been recognized that progestogens may have androgenic and estrogenic properties, and that the relative progestogenic, estrogenic and androgenic properties of synthetic progestogens are species-dependent. For example some 19-norethisterone progestogens have pronounced estrogenic properties in mice and rats but not in primates.

The influence of estrogen

The effect of progestogens on the female genital tract is also dependent on adequate estrogenic priming, but estrogens and progestogens act synergistically only in certain ratios, and the interaction is dependent on an optimal time sequence. Beier and colleagues demonstrated that the estrogen:progesterone ratio that is most favorable for the induction of endometrial decidualization lies in a more narrow band in primates compared to rats and dogs, and that this ratio is critical to the transformation[7]. It has also been demonstrated that the optimal estrogen:progesterone ratio is different, depending on the organ or the process under consideration; for example a ratio of 1:300 is optimal for mammogenesis in the rat, but the optimal ratio for a decidual reaction is 1:20 000[8]. Thus while the effect of each compound can vary, depending on the organ under consideration, it is also influenced by the presence of the other, further complicating attempts to study the biologic effects of combined preparations.

ASSESSMENT OF PROGESTOGENIC POTENCY

Receptor binding studies

As progestogens are defined by their ability to bind to the progesterone receptor, through which progesterone exerts its effect, tests have been designed to determine progestogenic potency by examining *in vitro* receptor binding affinity. Competitive binding assays are used for such tests, either in direct comparison with natural progesterone or with the progestogen reference compound R5020. The drawback of these methods is that they do not take into account the role of the intermediates which may themselves have receptor binding affinities. In the case of prodrugs such as norgestimate and desogestrel, the effect of the drug is primarily dependent on these metabolites, whilst less active metabolites may competitively bind to receptors, effecting a reduction of *in vivo* activity[9]. Furthermore, the results of such tests will be affected by experimental conditions such as temperature, period of incubation and animal species from which the cytosol preparation was obtained[10]. These drawbacks reduce the utility of receptor binding assays as surrogate indicators of *in vivo* action.

Bioassays

Bioassays, which rely on an assessment of the *in vivo* effects of administered steroids, overcome some of these difficulties but are hampered by the lack of organ or function specificity for steroids, and by the fact that many steroids and their metabolites may exert properties typical of other steroids or antagonists. The difficulty this creates in comparative studies is not to be underestimated, and although informative, any description of potency based on such tests will necessarily be an oversimplification. Bioassays for progestogenic potency were developed based on prominent and measurable influences such as their ability to inhibit uterine glandular proliferation or ovulation, to support the continuation of a pregnancy or to delay parturition in susceptible species. As mentioned above, the response of organs or tissues to a given steroid or to any particular dose is specific, which will be reflected in different estimates of potency depending on the bioassay used.

The Clauberg test, which is probably the most widely used bioassay for progesterone, is based on examining the effect of different doses of the test substance on estrogen-primed rabbit endometrium and determining the ability of the test substance to inhibit the proliferative influence and to induce secretory changes. However, endometrial morphologic and functional markers differ qualitatively as well as quantitatively depending on the nature of the administered progestogen[11]. Similar findings were reported in the human endometrium despite apparently different physiologic clinical effects[12,13]. Thus it becomes difficult, if not impossible, to determine a standard end-point for the assay that would describe progestogenic potency, and constructed dose–response curves may, therefore, not be comparable to each other[10].

The ability of administered progesterone to maintain pregnancy in rats following ovariectomy is the basis of the Pregnancy Maintenance test. Using this test, Edgren and colleagues argued that medroxyprogesterone acetate (MPA), norgestrel and LNG are active compounds, whereas norethynodrel and norethindrone are inactive[14]. This contrasts with the finding that norethisterone (NET) is as effective as progesterone based on the Delay of Parturition test[15], which, as its name suggests, is based on the ability of progestogens to delay parturition at term when administered to certain species. It is also interesting to note that whilst MPA appeared to be three times as potent as norgestrel based on the Clauberg test, it is only one-third as potent based on the Delay of Parturition test.

Tests of steroid potency in humans are based on the assessment of the effects of progesterone, such as its ability to delay menstruation (the Delay of Menstruation test), or to induce secretory endometrial changes either biochemical or morphologic.

The Delay of Menstruation test was originally described by Greenblatt and co-workers[16]. This test is based on the observation that the administration of an effective progestogen will delay withdrawal bleeding until 2–3 days after the treatment is discontinued. Based on this test it was estimated that NET and ethynodiol diacetate are twice as potent as NET acetate or MPA, and about five times as potent as norethynodrel. An important observation made by Pincus[17] during his pioneering field study of oral contraceptives in Puerto Rico, is that the removal of mestranol impurities from norethynodrel resulted in an increased incidence of breakthrough bleeding. This observation helped the evolution of the combined oral contraceptive pill, but it also demonstrated that the efficacy of progestogens in cycle control is affected by co-administration of estrogen. This was later confirmed using the Greenblatt test for all progestogens except MPA. More recently Habiba and colleagues suggested a possible link with hypo-estrogenism in the subset of women taking sequential combined HRT containing norethisterone acetate, in whom bleeding started before the end of tablet administration[18]. Thus the control of bleeding during HRT may not be solely dependent on the adequacy of the progestogenic component, as suggested by Padwick and colleagues[19].

Assessment of secretory changes in the endometrium

Various methods can be used for the assessment of secretory transformations induced by progestogens in the estrogen-primed endometrium. Direct assessment of biopsy material promises most accuracy, and studying the effect of steroids on the postmenopausal endometrium avoids the effect of endogenous menstrual cycle steroids (but not the postmenopausal milieu). The study by Whitehead and co-workers could be viewed in this context[3].

Whitehead and co-workers studied endometrial biopsies to compare the efficacy of NET in doses of 1, 2.5, 5 or 10 mg daily, and norgestrel in doses of 150 or 500 μg daily, to induce progestogenic changes in estrogen-primed postmenopausal endometrium. They also used the same approach to study the response longitudinally over 3, 6 and 10 days after the initiation of progestogen treatment. They studied morphological and ultrastructural and biochemical features, such as the ability of progestogens to suppress DNA synthesis, down-regulate the estrogen receptor, and increase the activity of the progestogen-sensitive enzymes estradiol dehydrogenase and isocitric dehydrogenase. The authors concluded that the use of 1 mg of NET or 150 μg of norgestrel achieved maximal suppression of DNA synthesis and near maximal reduction of nuclear estradiol receptor synthesis, and that the magnitude of this suppression was comparable to that achieved by 10 mg of NET or 500 µg norgestrel, or during the physiologic luteal phase. It is notable, however, that the levels of estradiol dehydrogenase and of isocitric dehydrogenase remained higher under the influence of the synthetic steroids compared with the physiologic cycle on day 6, at which time DNA synthesis and estrogen receptor production have both been suppressed.

This dissociation between the different 'progestogenic' influences echoes the case with animal bioassays, and will necessarily reduce the utility of these evaluations. The differential effects of steroids have also been shown to be time-dependent but not temporally related. It is also significant that the authors were unable to demonstrate a dose–effect relationship for biochemical parameters[3]. In a subsequent publication[20], the authors argued that based on their ability to suppress the estradiol receptor, 0.7 mg/day of NET, 150 µg/day of norgestrel, 20 mg/day of dydrogesterone and 300 mg/day of micronized progesterone are equivalent, and that LNG is eight times more potent than NET, which is about ten times more potent than MPA.

A recent study of postmenopausal HRT adopted a similar approach[21]. The authors undertook a dose-ranging study of the effect of oral trimegestone in a dose of 0.05, 0.1, 0.25 and 0.5 mg per day from days 15 to 28 with continuous micronized estradiol at a daily dose of 2 mg. They examined endometrial biopsies obtained on day 24 of the 28-day treatment cycle for the number of CD45[+], CD56[+] and CD3[+] leukocytes. However, there was no significant difference between the four treatment groups although they exhibited different bleeding patterns. The same authors found no histologic features that could discriminate between the four doses of trimegestone except for a reduced glandular secretion in the highest compared to the lower doses, despite a tenfold difference between the highest dose and the lowest[22]. These findings indicate the difficulties that are inherent in the *in vivo* assessment of progestogenic effects.

PROGESTOGENS IN COMBINATION WITH ESTROGENS

It has long been recognized that the administration of estrogen and progestogen can reproduce a regular menstrual cycle[23]. The importance of the relative amounts of both hormones was soon established[24]; for example, a high dose of estrogen can delay both menstruation and the development of secretory changes. Thus the development of secretory endometrial changes is dependent not only on the

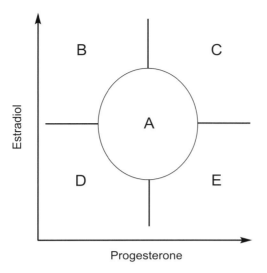

Figure 5.5. Endometrial histologic features related to the dose of administered estradiol and progesterone. A, secretory endometrium similar to that of the normal cycle; B, glands proliferated and dilated, epithelium pseudostratified, stroma underdeveloped; C, progesterone predominant, glands involuting, stroma predecidual; D, glands and stroma underdeveloped; E, glands underdeveloped, stroma predecidual. Reprinted (with modification) by permission from the American Society of Reproductive Medicine (Good RG, Moyer DL. *Fertil Steril* 1968;19:37–49)[28]

adequacy of the progestogenic challenge, but also on adequate estrogenic priming. One theory is that there is a certain threshold at which the endometrium can respond to progesterone[25]. It has also been suggested that maximal secretory transformation is dependent on the initial level of endometrial development[26,27]. This was demonstrated experimentally using the *Macaca mulatta* model[28], which showed that the normal menstrual cycle is dependent on an optimal dose of both estrogen and progesterone. Alterations in the administered dosage would result in the following changes (see Figure 5.5):

(1)	A suboptimal dose of estrogen and a suboptimal dose of progestogen result in glandular and stromal underdevelopment.

(2)	A suboptimal dose of estrogen and a high dose of progestogen result in underdeveloped glands and a predecidualized stroma.

(3)	A high dose of estrogen with a suboptimal dose of progestogen results in excessive glandular proliferation and dilatation and pseudostratification of the epithelium while the stroma remains underdeveloped.

(4) A high dose of estrogen and a high dose of progestogen result in involution of the glands and stromal predecidualization.

(5) Shortening or prolongation of the length of the proliferative phase had no influence on endometrial histology in biopsies taken during the luteal phase.

(6) The absolute amount is more important for an optimum response than the ratio between the two hormones.

EFFECT OF HRT ON THE ENDOMETRIUM

Assessment of endometrial morphologic features in postmenopausal women who experienced regular bleeding while using a cyclical sequential combined HRT containing norethisterone demonstrated significant differences when compared to the physiologic cycle[12]. Histologic features differed both quantitatively and qualitatively, which is in agreement with studies of the endometrium under the influence of the combined oral contraceptive pill[29].

Habiba and colleagues demonstrated that the glandular component in HRT-stimulated endometrium exhibited a mixture of features some, but not all, of which are represented in the early, mid- or late luteal phase[12]. The stroma exhibited relatively more advanced features, i.e. glandular and stromal dyssynchrony. The study also demonstrated dissociation between the classical histologic features and the occurrence of bleeding. This dissociation between morphology and function raises important questions concerning the utility of traditional histologic classification in the assessment of the different states of the endometrium under HRT, and the use of functional parameters (e.g. bleeding) as an index of endometrial changes. Furthermore, the study of functional and structural markers in the endometrium under the influence of HRT also demonstrated significant differences when compared to the physiologic cycle[12]. Expression of α smooth muscle action protein (αSMA) around the glands and in the stroma is higher under HRT stimulation, which indicates a persistent follicular phase feature, and/or tissue remodeling or stress, which, in turn, could be characteristic of the progestogen used. The expression of other functional markers such as β-lactoglobulin (α_2-PEG), heat-shock protein 27 (Hsp27), estrogen receptor (ER) and progesterone receptor (PR), also demonstrated the dissimilarity between endometrium under the effects of HRT and that of the natural cycle[13]. Glandular epithelium on HRT expressed lower levels of β-lactoglobulin (the most abundant endometrial secretory protein) compared to the mid- and late luteal phases, but higher levels compared to the early luteal phase, and expressed the same level of PR compared to the mid- and late luteal phases but lower levels compared to the early luteal phase.

Effect of progestogen on the ultrastructural features of the endometrium

During the proliferative phase the endometrium exhibits ultrastructural evidence of increased protein synthesis which accompanies cellular proliferation, for example an increase in free and bound ribosomes, mitochondria, Golgi bodies and primary lysosomes in both the glands and the stroma. Under the influence of progesterone during the luteal phase, ribosomes increase in number and the rough endoplasmic reticulum develops. Another feature that becomes apparent on electron microscopy is the nuclear (nucleolar) channel system (NCS) of seven sets of three-branched tubules connected to the nuclear membrane. This system is characteristic of the postovulatory uterine epithelium in the human and is detected between days 18 and 25 of the cycle, being maximally developed between days 19 and 21[30].

Studies using luteinizing hormone (LH)-surge dated endometrial biopsies have shown that the structural changes in the glandular epithelium during the first 6 days of the secretory phase are precisely regulated with small inter-individual variation[24,31,32]. The NCS was also shown to be related to ovulation and absent in users of progesterone intrauterine contraceptive devices (IUCDs) or the minipill, but present in the endometrium after estrogen and progesterone treatment in *in vitro* fertilization (IVF) cycles[26]. Such findings would suggest that ultrastructural changes could be useful markers for progestogenic potency. However, the development of the NCS system is not a prerequisite for secretory activity, and was shown to be a function of the type of progesterone and of the adequacy of the initial estrogenic priming. Progesterone, chlormadinone and MPA, but not 19-nortestosterone derivatives, produce the NCS[30]; 19-nortestosterone derivatives induce giant mitochondria and glycogen deposits[33].

The heterogeneity of response demonstrated in these studies renders the use of endometrial development and/or differentiation in the assessment of progestogenic potency less adequate than might be hoped. However, analysis of the results should also take into account the fact that progestogens have some properties (e.g. androgenic effect) that are different from those of progesterone, and it could be that these antagonize the progestogenic potency, for example β-lactoglobulin expression and the incomplete suppression of PR[13]. Our understanding of the effects of androgenic steroids on the endometrium is, however, limited and to date no work has directly compared the effects of androgenic and non-androgenic steroids, although it appears from published work that many similarities exist in the histologic features linked to all synthetic steroids.

ANDROGENIC POTENCY

Androgenic potency is a recognized property of some progestogens, particularly those related to testosterone. Androgen receptor binding assays and bioassays have been used to assess the androgenic properties of progestogens, in an analogous fashion to the use of progesterone receptor binding assays (similar assays are also used for estrogens). These are necessarily associated with the same difficulties as tests for progestogenic potency. In humans, assessment of androgenic properties is commonly based on the ability of androgens to suppress sex hormone-binding globulin (SHBG). But comparative studies have only been carried out in pre-menopausal women in relation to the use of oral contraceptives; therefore the results will necessarily reflect the interaction between the estrogenic and the progestogenic components of the oral contraceptive pill, balanced against the influence of the administered agent on ovarian steroid production.

MECHANISM OF ACTION OF SEX STEROIDS

Sex steroids exert their effects through interaction with their receptors, and progestogens with estrogenic or androgenic properties exert their effects through their (or their metabolites') binding with the corresponding receptor[34]. Estrogen receptors are members of a large superfamily of nuclear receptors functioning as ligand-activated transcription factors. A different mechanism for estrogen action, where receptors have not been localized within target genes, involves the activation of AP-1 sites, following activation of c-*jun* and c-*fos* genes[35]. It has been suggested that steps downstream of DNA binding may be responsible for distinguishing between agonist- and antagonist-activated receptors[36]. More recently it has been demonstrated that ligands activating the AP-1 site induce a differential stimulatory or inhibitory effect depending on the type of receptor (ERα or ERβ)[37]. For example, at the AP-1 site 17β-estradiol stimulates transcription with ERα, but inhibits transcription with ERβ. The effects of anti-estrogens also vary depending on the receptor type[37]. Whether estrogenic steroids have a differential effect on

ERα, ERβ, or on the AP-1 site is not known, but it is possible that a differential effect exists that may be linked to different expressed phenotypes. Besides receptor-mediated properties, some of the effects of estrogen may be exerted directly on the cell membrane[38,39], or through the mediation of stimulatory or inhibitory second messengers[40]. There is some evidence for progestogens being converted to estrogens, albeit in small quantities. One study estimated that norethisterone administered in large doses to postmenopausal women is converted to ethinylestradiol at a conversion ratio of between 0.4 and 0.7%. The rate of conversion suggests that the dose of norethisterone commonly used in HRT (1 mg) would add 4 μg of ethinylestradiol[41].

Androgen receptors (AR) have been demonstrated in the endometrial stroma but not the epithelium[42], and it is possible that these mediate the androgenic properties of progestogens. The level of AR has been shown to be lower during the late follicular phase and to be absent during the late luteal phase of the natural cycle[42]. AR level is under the influence of dihydrotestosterone (DHT). In the natural cycle it is possible that the competition between progesterone and testosterone for 5α-reductase results in diminished DHT and inhibition of AR level. Whether norethisterone exerts a similar effect is not known, but norethisterone (and possibly its metabolites) have an androgen-like potency, which is reduced by 5α-reductase.

The menopause itself is a hyperandrogenic state with a higher level of circulating androstenedione, testosterone and dehydroepiandrosterone, and may thus be associated with a relative abundance of AR. However, in the absence of data on the effects of AR stimulation on endometrial structure and function it remains unknown to what degree the androgenic potency of progestogens contributes to features observed in the endometrium (Figure 5.6).

Progesterone exerts its progestogenic effect on the endometrium through interaction with the PR, although direct membrane effects have also been reported[43]. The effect of progesterone is dependent on estrogenic influences and on growth factors such as insulin-like growth factor, and epidermal growth factor (EGF), as well as on the interaction with the PR, which involves other proteins such as Hsp70 and Hsp90. Progestogens may also have anti-progestogenic effects, particularly when given in large doses, e.g. norethisterone in large doses together with its metabolites (5α-dihydronorethisterone and 3β,5α-tetrahydronorethisterone) has been shown to exhibit receptor-mediated antiprogestational and anti-implantation effects similar to those of RU486[44,45]. The different effects of progestogens compared to progesterone cannot be explained solely by their relative binding

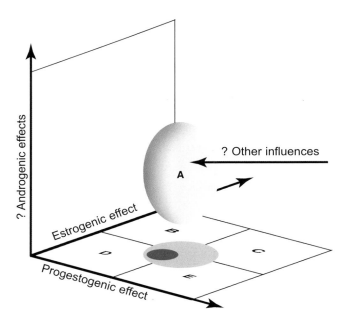

Figure 5.6. A three-dimensional model depicting the factors, besides estrogen and progestogen, that may be relevant to endometrial differentiation. A, secretory endometrium similar to that of the normal cycle; B, glands proliferated and dilated, epithelium pseudo-stratified, stroma underdeveloped; C, progesterone predominant, glands involuting, stroma predecidual; D, glands and stroma underdeveloped; E, glands underdeveloped, stroma predecidual. Modified from the two-dimensional model shown in Figure 5.5

affinity (RBA) to the PR, as both norethisterone and MPA exhibited stronger glycogen induction compared to progesterone, although compared to progesterone, norethisterone had a weaker, and MPA a stronger RBA[46].

THE PLACE OF PHARMACOKINETICS

The many proposed definitions of bioavailability underscore some of the difficulties encountered with the use of the term. The term has been variably defined with reference to a number of variables: (1) the amount of drug absorbed, (2) the total serum level of the progestogen, (3) the proportion of the drug in an active form, (4) the amount of active drug reaching the effector sites and (5) the rate of absorption[47]. Differences in steroid metabolism, the activity of the metabolites and the level of circulating metabolites are just a few of the factors that complicate studies of steroid bioavailability. Clearly, biologic activity is affected by bioavailability, but other factors such as affinity to receptors, and the rates of metabolism and elimination play an important role. Biologic activity may also depend on post-absorption metabolism. Examples include the metabolism of desogestrel into its active metabolite 3-ketodesogestrel, or the conversion of norgestimate into LNG, both of which mainly take place in the liver. Parenteral administration is associated with difficulties related to the specific route of absorption. Further difficulties arise because drug absorption is affected not only by individual or generic factors, but also by features typical of the particular formulation – which may be characteristic of the manufacturing process itself. Examples of these include the presence of excipients or the process of micronization, both of which facilitate absorption. Thus bioavailability may differ according to the method of preparation, and as such ought not to be considered as typical of the particular chemical compound under consideration.

The above indicates that the utility of bioavailability studies in determining biologic activity of progestogens would necessarily be limited. Indeed the scarcity of studies on drugs such as MPA and norgestimate has not precluded their use. Wide variability has been reported in serum concentration after oral administration of progestogens, e.g. norethisterone concentration was reported to vary by a factor of 9 after oral administration, and the serum half-life ranged from 6.1 to 12.3 hours[48], and no studies have attempted to correlate such variability with clinical behavior, for example the efficacy of the oral contraceptive pill, or with end-organ response.

CONCLUSION

This chapter explores current understanding of the methods used in the assessment of the effects of administered progestogens on endometrial differentiation, and the difficulties inherent in available techniques. The discussion highlights many areas where further research is needed to unravel the complexities of interactions and the heterogeneity of end-organ response. Much less is known about the effects of steroids on other steroid-sensitive organs, which will necessarily be different from the effects on the endometrium. But being more accessible, the endometrium serves as a useful model for research.

REFERENCES

1. Smith D, Prentice R, Thompson D, Herrman W. Association of exogenous estrogen and endometrial carcinoma. *N Engl J Med* 1975;293:1164–7
2. Ziel HK, Finkle WD. Increased risk of endometrial carcinoma among users of conjugated estrogens. *N Engl J Med* 1975;293:1167–70
3. Whitehead MI, Townsend PT, Pryse-Davies J, *et al.* Effects of estrogens and progestins on the biochemistry and morphology of the postmenopausal endometrium. *N Engl J Med* 1981;305:1599–605
4. Creasy GW, Kafrissen ME, Upmalis D. Review of the endometrial effects of estrogens and progestins. *Obstet Gynecol Surv* 1992;47:654–78
5. Birch AJ. Hydroaromatic steroid hormones. *J Chem Soc* 1950;1:367–8
6. Robbins A, Bardin CW. Nestorone progestin. The ideal progestin for use in controlled release delivery systems. *Ann N Y Acad Sci* 1997;828:38–46
7. Beier S, Duterberg B, El-Etreby MF, *et al.* Toxicology of hormonal fertility regulating agents. In Benagiano G, Diczfalusy E, eds. *Pharmacological Modulation of Steroid Action.* New York: Raven Press, 1983:261–346
8. El-Etreby MF, Beier S, Gunzel P. Comparative endocrine pharmacodynamics of contraceptive steroids. In Michal F, ed. *Safety Requirements for Contraceptive Steroids.* Cambridge: Cambridge University Press, 1989:179–92
9. Juchem M, Pollow K. Binding of oral contraceptive progestogens to serum proteins and cytoplasmic receptor. *Am J Obstet Gynecol* 1990;163:2171–83
10. Larsson KS, Machin D. Predictability of the safety of hormonal contraceptives from canine toxicological studies. In Michal F, ed. *Safety Requirements for Contraceptive Steroids.* Cambridge: Cambridge University Press, 1989:230–69
11. Edgren RA. Progestogens. In Givens JR, ed. *Clinical Use of Sex Steroids.* Chicago: Year Book Medical Publishers, 1980:1–29
12. Habiba MA, Bell SC, Al-Azzawi F. Endometrial responses to hormone replacement therapy: histological features compared with those of late luteal phase endometrium. *Hum Reprod* 1988;13:1674–82
13. Habiba MA, Bell SC, Al-Azzawi F. The effect of hormone replacement therapy on the immunoreactive concentrations in the endometrium of oestrogen and progesterone receptor, heat shock protein 27, and human beta-lactoglobulin. *Hum Reprod* 2000;15:36–42
14. Edgren RA, Jones RC, Peterson DL. A biological classification of progestational agents. *Fertil Steril* 1967;18:238–56
15. Edgren RA, Peterson DL. Delay of parturition in rats by various progestational steroids. *Proc Soc Exp Biol Med* 1966;123:867–9
16. Greenblatt RB, Jungck EC, Barfield WE. A new test of efficacy of progestational compounds. *Ann N Y Acad Sci* 1958;71:717
17. Diczfaluzy E. Gregory Pincus and steroidal contraception. A new departure into the history of mankind. *J Steroid Biochem* 1979;11:3–11
18. Habiba MA, Bell SC, Abrams K, Al-Azzawi F. Endometrial responses to hormone replacement therapy: the bleeding pattern. *Hum Reprod* 1996;11:503–8
19. Padwick M, Pryse-Davies J, Whitehead M. A simple method for determining the optimal dosage of progestin in postmenopausal women receiving estrogens. *N Engl J Med* 1986;315:930–4

20. King RJ, Whitehead MI. Assessment of the potency of orally administered progestins in women. *Fertil Steril* 1986;46:1062–6

21. Wahab M, Thompson J, Al-Azzawi F. The distribution of endometrial leukocytes and their proliferation markers in trimegestone-treated postmenopausal women compared to the endometrium of the natural cycle: a dose-ranging study. *Hum Reprod* 1999;14:1201–6

22. Wahab M, Thompson J, Hamid B, *et al*. Endometrial histomorphometry of trimegestone-based sequential hormone replacement therapy: a weighted comparison with the endometrium of the natural cycle. *Hum Reprod* 1999;14:2609–18

23. Kaufmann C. Echte menstruelle blutung bei kastrierten frauen nach zufuhr von follikel- und corpus luteum-hormon. *Klin Wochenschr* 1933;12:217

24. Ferin J, Schilkker E. Artificial cycles in oophorectomized women. *Int J Fertil* 1960;5:19

25. Johannisson E, Landgren BM, Rohr HP, Diczfalusy E. Endometrial morphology and peripheral hormone levels in women with regular menstrual cycles. *Fertil Steril* 1987; 48:401–8

26. Dockery P, Tidey RR, Li TC, Cooke ID. A morphometric study of the uterine glandular epithelium in women with premature ovarian failure undergoing hormone replacement therapy. *Hum Reprod* 1991;6:1354–64

27. Li TC, Dockery P, Cooke ID. Effect of exogenous progesterone administration on the morphology of normally developing endometrium in the pre-implantation period. *Hum Reprod* 1991;6:641–4

28. Good RG, Moyer DL. Estrogen–progesterone relationships in the development of secretory endometrium. *Fertil Steril* 1968;19:37–49

29. Dallenbach-Hellweg G. *Histopathology of the Endometrium*, 4th edn. Berlin: Springer-Verlag, 1987:166–86

30. Spornitz UM. The functional morphology of the human endometrium and decidua. *Adv Anat Embryol Cell Biol* 1992;124:1–99

31. Dockery P, Li TC, Rogers AW, *et al*. The ultrastructure of the glandular epithelium in the timed endometrial biopsy. *Hum Reprod* 1988;3:826–34

32. Dockery P, Rogers AW. The effects of steroids on the fine structure of the endometrium. *Baillière's Clin Obstet Gynaecol* 1989;3:227–48

33. Kohorn EI, Rice SI, Hemperly S, Gordon M. The relation of the structure of progestational steroids to nucleolar differentiation in human endometrium. *J Clin Endocrinol Metab* 1972;34:257–64

34. Oropeza MV, Campos MG, Lemus AE, *et al*. Estrogenic actions of norethisterone and its A-ring reduced metabolites. Induction of *in vitro* uterine sensitivity to serotonin. *Arch Med Res* 1994;25:307–10

35. Alkhalaf M, Murphy LC. Regulation of c-jun and jun-B by progestins in T-47D human breast cancer cells. *Mol Endocrinol* 1992;6:1625–33

36. McDonnell DP, Lieberman BA, Norris J. Development of tissue selective estrogen receptor modulators. In Baird DT, Schutz G, Krattenmacher R, eds. *Organ-selective Actions of Steroid Hormones*. Schering Research Foundation Workshop 16. Berlin: Springer-Verlag, 1995:1–28

37. Paech K, Webb P, Kuiper GG, *et al*. Differential ligand activation of estrogen receptors ERalpha and ERbeta at AP1 sites. *Science* 1997;277:1508–10

38. Tuohimaa P, Blauer M, Pasanen S, *et al*. Mechanisms of action of sex steroid hormones: basic concepts and clinical correlations. *Maturitas* 1996;23:S3–12

39. Collins P, Webb C. Estrogen hits the surface. *Nature Med* 1999;5:1130–1
40. Bern HA. Is estrogen a cellular signal controlling uterine function? In Lavia LA, ed. *Cellular Signals Controlling Uterine Function*. New York: Plenum Press, 1991:5–9
41. Kuhnz W, Heuner A, Humpel M, *et al. In vivo* conversion of norethisterone and norethisterone acetate to ethinyl estradiol in postmenopausal women. *Contraception* 1997; 56:379–85
42. Mertens HJ, Heineman MJ, Koudstaal J, *et al.* Androgen receptor content in human endometrium. *Eur J Obstet Gynecol Reprod Biol* 1996;70:11–13
43. Schumacher M. Rapid membrane effects of steroid hormones: an emerging concept in neuroendocrinology. *Trends Neurosci* 1990;13:359–62
44. Castro I, Cerbon MA, Pasapera AM, *et al.* Molecular mechanisms of the antihormonal and antiimplantation effects of norethisterone and its A-ring reduced metabolites. *Mol Reprod Dev* 1995;40:157–63
45. Pasapera AM, Cerbon MA, Castro I, *et al.* Norethisterone metabolites modulate the uteroglobin and progesterone receptor gene expression in prepubertal rabbits. *Biol Reprod* 1995;52:426–32
46. Shapiro SS, Dyer RD, Colas AE. Synthetic progestins: *in vitro* potency on human endometrium and specific binding to cytosol receptor. *Am J Obstet Gynecol* 1978;132: 549–54
47. Fotherby K. Bioavailability of orally administered sex steroids used in oral contraception and hormone replacement therapy. *Contraception* 1996;54:59–69
48. Back DJ, Breckenridge AM, Crawford FE, *et al.* Kinetics of norethindrone in women. I. Radioimmunoassay and concentrations during multiple dosing. *Clin Pharmacol Ther* 1978;24:439–47

6

Endometrial histology under the effect of sex steroids: the contribution of histomorphometry

M. Wahab

INTRODUCTION

The endometrium responds to the ovarian cycle of folliculogenesis, ovulation and corpus luteum formation by undergoing cyclical growth and differentiation in preparation for the implantation of the blastocyst. If implantation does not occur, the corpus luteum degenerates and the endometrium responds by shedding its functionalis layers. This involves a series of events which resemble an acute inflammatory process, followed by healing. It is remarkable, however, that tissue repair and healing in the endometrium occurs in the absence of scarring.

The fluctuating levels of sex steroids generated during the ovarian cycle are influenced by a variety of innate and environmental factors, such that the levels of these substances are not exactly replicated from cycle to cycle and are certainly not identical between women. The corollary is that such variables may themselves be responsible for variations in the length of the natural menstrual cycle, its rhythm and even the amount of blood loss. Furthermore, endometrial growth and differentiation are variable within the endometrial cavity itself[1,2]. In addition, the parameters used in assigning phase development to the endometrial sample are applicable to the functionalis layer, and fragments of the basalis layer incorporated in such samples are, therefore, undatable.

The variability of endometrial histology during the natural cycle profoundly influences the diagnosis of the stage of development and fosters a highly subjective assessment of it. Not surprisingly, therefore, the clinical management of functional disorders of the menstrual cycle has not been helped to any significant extent by routine histologic characterization of the endometrium. A trend has evolved in clinical tradition to ignore neoplastic changes of the endometrium, consequently tempting both pathologists and gynecologists alike to declare such tissue samples to be benign and relegating the condition to the category of 'functional menstrual disorders' with concomitant empirical management.

The aims of this chapter are to illustrate the classical histologic description of the endometrium in specified phases of the natural cycle, to describe the reported changes in the endometrium that result from exogenous sex steroid therapy, and to present a method of evaluating the impact of individual histologic parameters on the final diagnosis of a particular phase of endometrial development. Most workers in this field accept the detailed descriptions of endometrial development during the natural cycle given by Noyes and colleagues[3] and Dallenbach-Hellweg and Poulsen[4].

HISTOLOGY OF THE ENDOMETRIUM

Endometrial healing following menstruation is usually complete by day 5 post-menstruum. This is followed by a phase of growth under the effect of estrogen, which quantitatively dominates the endocrine milieu until ovulation occurs (Figure 6.1)[3,4].

The proliferative phase

Owing to the overlap of the histologic characteristics and the inter-observer variations between pathologists[5], dating the endometrium accurately in this phase may prove difficult, although, somewhat arbitrarily, early, mid- and late proliferative phases are usually described.

Early proliferative phase (days 4–7)
The glands are straight and narrow and evenly distributed in a loose stroma. The luminal epithelium is flat and the stromal cells have small dense nuclei in sparse cytoplasm.

Mid-proliferative phase (days 8–11)
There are increases in glandular tortuosity and glandular epithelial mitoses and the luminal epithelium is starting to become columnar.

Late proliferative phase (days 12–14)

Glandular tortuosity is markedly increased, with the lining of the epithelium showing pseudostratification and prominent mitoses. The luminal epithelium is now columnar and stroma cells exhibit frequent mitoses.

The luteal phase

Following ovulation corpus luteum formation has an intense steroidogenetic role. The resulting spectrum of steroids is responsible for modulating stimuli for differentiation and other preparatory changes in anticipation of implantation. Quantitatively, the main steroids synthesized are estradiol and progesterone. The luteal phase usually lasts for 14 days and histologic dating of endometrial responses depends on the changes observed in the glandular epithelium during the first week following ovulation, such as mitoses, pseudostratification, subnuclear vacuolation, with subsequent translocation to the supranuclear position, and finally intra-glandular secretion. Changes in the stroma characterize the second week following ovulation and are mainly those of stromal edema, mitoses, predecidual reaction and leukocyte infiltration[2–4].

These changes start 36–48 hours following ovulation:

(1) Day 2: basal vacuoles appear in the glandular epithelium, and the epithelial nuclei form a single row;

(2) Day 4: a small rim of mucopolysaccharides can be observed at the luminal margin of glandular epithelial cells;

(3) Day 5: the majority of the nuclei have returned to the base of the glandular epithelium, with supranuclear vacuoles;

(4) Day 7: the glandular lumen is filled with glycogen and there is patchy development of stromal edema, which reaches its maximum on the 8th day;

(5) Day 9: stromal edema starts to subside and glandular secretion ceases; and

(6) Day 10: the endometrium shows two distinct layers, the upper, compact layer consisting mainly of stromal cells where predecidual changes develop, and a lower layer of distended tortuous glands.

The height of the endometrium starts to regress by the 12th day. T lymphocytes, mast cells and polymorphonuclear granulocytes appear in the premenstrual endometrium.

a

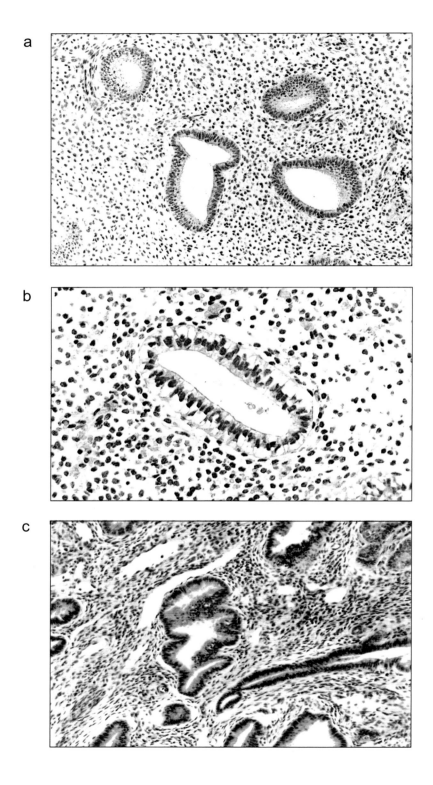

b

c

d

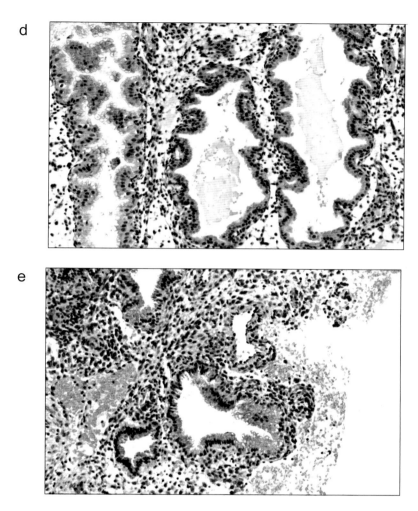

e

Figure 6.1. Histology (hematoxylin and eosin (H&E) stain) of the endometrium through the natural cycle. (**a**) Proliferative phase (original magnification × 200); (**b**) early luteal phase, showing glandular subnuclear vacuoles (original magnification × 400); (**c**) and (**d**) mid- and late luteal phases, showing glandular tortuosity and secretions (original magnification × 200); (**e**) menstrual phase, showing tissue disintegration (original magnification × 200)

The menstrual phase

On days 13 and 14 postovulation the endometrium shows evidence of dissociation of glands and stroma, together with patchy hemorrhages in the superficial layer, while the basal part remains intact[4].

ENDOMETRIAL EFFECT OF EXOGENOUS SEX STEROID THERAPY

Exogenous sex steroids administered for contraception may influence endometrial growth by the suppression of steroidogenesis together with the provision of constant amounts of the steroids. These agents induce a relatively thin endometrium, which is shed as a result of steroid withdrawal in the pill-free week. Incomplete ovarian suppression in premenopausal women using contraceptive steroids may result in intermenstrual bleeding, and as such may be successfully managed by increasing the dose of estrogen. However, the administration of the combined oral contraceptive pill for extended periods – that is, without interruption – may well delay the onset of bleeding, but bleeding will eventually occur. This also suggests that instability of the endometrium can be independent of the concurrent dose of the sex steroids being administered.

The advent of the progestogen-only pill or minipill for contraception introduced a different endometrial behavior, in which the continued administration of low doses of a progestogen, not enough to cause ovarian suppression, offsets the stimulatory effects on endometrial growth of endogenous estrogens. The incidence of endometrial instability, and consequently poor cycle control, is high.

Changes observed in endometrial glands and stroma

The effects of contraceptive steroids on endometrial histology depend on the type, dose and duration of the steroid administered. Oral norethisterone (NET), 300 µg/day given as a contraceptive for 3 months, reduces significantly the number and diameter of endometrial glands[6]. Administered at 50 µg/day through a vaginal ring, NET does not affect the size or number of glands per unit area, but when the dose is increased to 200 µg/day it significantly reduces the size of the individual glands at 6 weeks, and reduces the number of these glands if given for 10 weeks[6].

Prolonged exposure to a levonorgestrel (LNG)-releasing vaginal device is associated with a significant decrease in glandular number and diameter and an increase in glandular and stromal mitoses during the treatment period[7]. An LNG-laden intravaginal ring delivering a dose of 10 µg/day has no effect on the endometrial glands, but in a dose of 20 µg/day for 6 weeks it is associated with a reduction in glandular diameter, while a reduction in glandular size is documented when the dose is increased to 25 µg/day for 6–10 weeks of treatment[6]. On the other hand, subdermally administered LNG (Norplant®, Aventis Pharma, UK) given for 12 months is associated with a suppressed endometrium, that is small glands with exhausted secretion, and edematous stroma with predecidual transformation[8].

Other changes attributed to the administration of progestogens include arrested secretions, a condition that has been described following 3 months of progestogen use; here proliferation of the endometrial glands is arrested, probably owing to down-regulation of glandular estrogen receptors as a direct effect of the progestogen, particularly when progestogen is administered in high doses. The glands are sparse and lined by atrophic epithelium. If treatment continues for 6 months, arrested secretion may change to fibrous atrophy. The glands almost disappear, while the stromal cells are small and spindle-shaped[4]. The effects of parenteral depot progestogens can last for months after cessation of their use. The pattern of changes induced with progestogen treatment includes decidual (pregnancy-like), secretory and atrophic changes, although there is usually an overlap between these various patterns.

Changes observed in endometrial vasculature

Exogenous sex steroids modify the vascular architecture of the endometrium; the use of Norplant is associated with increased microvascular density compared to controls[9], while oral medroxyprogesterone acetate (MPA) or NET for 5–6 months has been associated with reduced vascular density and an increased number of dilated venules[10]. A similar finding was reported using an LNG-releasing intra-uterine contraceptive device (IUCD)[11]. NET administered orally in a cyclical sequential hormone replacement therapy (HRT) regimen with estradiol for 3 months was associated with a higher number of small vascular spaces compared to either the endometrium of the natural cycle or to the effect of the norpregnane progestogen trimegestone administered as a sequential combined HRT regimen with estradiol[12].

ENDOMETRIAL MORPHOMETRY

The endocrine effect on the endometrium has for many years been subjectively assessed, using criteria laid down by Noyes and colleagues[3] and others[4]. These criteria are well suited for establishing the diagnosis of a particular phase of the menstrual cycle. Nevertheless interobserver variation, even among experienced histopathologists, has been shown to be high[13]. Furthermore, the effects of contraceptive steroids on the endometrium are not uniform.

Most studies of endometrial morphometry under the effect of exogenous sex steroids suffer from a small sample size and short duration of treatment or an unclear method of assessment. Johannisson and co-workers[14] studied the effects of LNG administered through a vaginal ring as a contraceptive for 90 days. LNG significantly reduced the glandular diameter, glandular volume density and the number of the arterioles in the endometrial tissue[14]. However it is not clear how the last conclusion was reached since there is no mention of the method of assessment of endometrial vascularity. In addition, measurements per 1000 glandular cells[15] or volume density of the stroma[14] are not uniform entities, since 1000 glandular cells may involve 10 or even 20 glands, and these may occupy larger or smaller areas of the specimen, depending on the glandular size. Ludwig studied the morphologic changes associated with different progestogens and for different durations of treatment; however in this study there was only one patient in each group[16].

There is a paucity in the literature of articles describing the histologic changes associated with HRT in postmenopausal women. Casanas-Roux's group studied the morphometric characteristics associated with oral estrogen and cyclically administered progesterone vaginal gel and found an increase in glandular coiling in response to this regimen that mimicked the glandular changes in the luteal phase[17]. Other reports included a single point assessment of each histologic parameter, and therefore did not address the significance of the contribution of other parameters to the overall picture of the samples[18].

Data management of endometrial histomorphometry

Given that the subjectivity arising in routine histologic assessment of the endometrium does not lend itself to quantitative assessment of these changes observed with the different treatment regimens, and that comparisons limited to single parameters may well miss the overall state of development of the endometrium, a comprehensive approach to the whole set of measurable indices is required. Therefore a mathematical model, which includes all these histologic parameters evaluated per unit area, is needed in order to compare the differing effects of different sex steroids on the endometrium and relate such changes to those observed during the natural cycle.

Linear discriminant analysis (LDA) is a suitable method for evaluating these changes in a tissue as highly variable as the endometrium. LDA is a statistical method whereby weighted combinations of the measurements are sought that best separate different groups of samples. By identifying those measurements which have the largest standardized weights it is possible to identify and quantify which variables reliably distinguish between the groups, or phases of development. The measurements are standardized by subtracting the overall mean from the individual observation value and dividing the difference by the pooled within-group standard deviations, so that the effects of the scale of measurement are removed and the relative contributions of the different measurements are more clearly seen[19].

In an attempt to illustrate the concept of linear discriminant analysis as a means of evaluating the contribution of individual histologic parameters to the overall diagnostic picture, we utilized histologic specimens obtained during the natural cycle. These specimens were characterized by the date of the last menstrual period, days post-luteinizing hormone (LH) surge and an independent assessment by two histopathologists, and only when all agreed on a particular phase of endometrial development were the samples included in the study. An image analysis program was used to capture histologic images and measure specified parameters of these tissues. The following were assessed:

(1)   Glands: total glandular area, average glandular diameter, number of complete and incomplete glands per field, glandular epithelial height in the glands (columnar or cuboidal), regularity of the glandular epithelial surface (smooth or irregular), percentage of gland containing luminal secretions and subnuclear vacuoles, and number of glandular invaginations (telescoping) in the field.

(2)   Vascularity was examined for total vascular space area, average vascular space diameter and number of vascular spaces per field.

(3)   Stromal cellular density was assessed by counting the nuclei.

The main results of the study

The total glandular area increased significantly in the luteal phase compared to the proliferative phase ($p < 0.004$), but there was no difference in the number of glands, while glandular epithelial height was lowest in the mid-luteal phase but became taller as the endometrium advanced in the luteal and menstrual phases. There was a statistically significantly higher number of glands with vacuoles in the early luteal phase compared to the other phases of the natural cycle ($p < 0.004$), while glandular secretions were different across the phases of the cycle but more abundant in mid- and late luteal phases. Total vascular space area increased as the luteal phase advanced, and was highest in the menstrual phase ($p < 0.05$), but there was no difference in the mean number of the vascular spaces.

Linear discriminant functions

It is possible to have more than one linear discriminant function, depending on the different planes in which we are trying to analyze the data to distinguish between the phases of the natural cycle[19]. The first linear discriminant function showed most discrimination, followed by the second, third, etc. The signs and sizes of the standardized weights corresponded to the importance of each variable to the final score (Table 6.1). The mean total glandular area contributed highly to the score of linear discriminant function 1, while the second linear discriminant function was dominated by a higher percentage of glands with vacuolation or telescoping, lower mean vascular space area, and lower percentage of glands with columnar epithelial

Table 6.1. Standardized weights assigned to individual histologic parameters along the first four linear discriminant functions. Data from Wahab M, Thompson J, Hamid B, *et al. Hum Reprod* 1999;14:2609–18[19]

Histologic parameters	Linear discriminant functions			
	1	*2*	*3*	*4*
% glandular area	1.19	0.37	−0.75	0.25
% vascular space area	−0.34	−1.02	0.34	−0.19
Average glandular diameter	−0.51	−0.12	−0.10	−0.62
Average vascular space diameter	0.38	0.13	−0.11	−0.30
Stromal cell count	0.14	−0.01	−0.25	−0.09
No. of complete glands	−0.29	−0.27	0.34	−0.14
No. of 'half' glands	0.15	0.14	0.59	0.13
% gland with columnar lining	−0.06	−0.46	0.78	0.13
No. of vascular spaces	0.21	0.20	−0.11	0.49
% gland with vacuoles	0.37	0.68	0.01	−0.53
% gland with secretions	−0.02	−0.33	−0.27	0.78
% gland with telescoping	−0.00	0.51	0.11	0.08
% gland with smooth surface	0.33	−0.14	−0.30	−0.12

lining (Figure 6.2a). If Figure 6.2a is rotated clockwise then Figure 6.2b results. The rotated linear discriminant functions depend most critically on just a few variables (Table 6.2)[19]. If only the variables with standardized coefficients greater than 0.4 are used then new discriminant functions are obtained that capture most of the discriminatory information in this data set (Figure 6.2c).

Using the original raw data of the histologic parameters assessed to reconstruct a new Figure 6.2c, the following expressions can be used to assign a value for the first and second linear discriminant functions, where they can be compared to the different phases of the natural cycle:

$$\text{first ldf} = 0.139(A) + 0.797(B) \qquad\qquad \text{I}$$
$$\text{second ldf} = 0.127(A) - 0.909(B) - 0.029(C) + 0.061(D) + 0.019(E) \qquad \text{II}$$

where first ldf = first linear discriminant function; second ldf = second linear discriminant function; A = mean percentage total glandular area; B = mean percentage total vascular space area; C = average glandular diameter; D = average vascular space diameter; and E = percentage of glands with vacuolation.

We utilized the LDA to study the histologic changes under the effect of a new nor-pregnane progestogen, trimegestone, given to postmenopausal women in one of four doses (0.05, 0.1, 0.25 and 0.5 mg/day) from day 15 to day 28, in combination with estradiol 2 mg as a cyclical sequential regimen. The histologic changes induced by trimegestone were similar regardless of the dose (Figure 6.2a)[20], in contrast to the bleeding patterns induced in the women who participated in this study, which differed according to the dosage of trimegestone[20,21].

The first linear discriminant function distinguishes the luteal phases from trimegestone-treated endometrium, and the second linear discriminant function distinguishes between the trimegestone group and the proliferative, menstrual and mid-luteal phases (Figure 6.2a). The first rotated linear discriminant function distinguishes between the trimegestone and the phases of the natural cycle, while the second distinguishes clearly between phases of the natural cycle (Figure 6.2b).

The evaluation of endometrial histologic data using this method clearly separate this HRT regimen (or any regimen to be tested) from the other phases of the natural cycle and helps to quantify the differences between the samples and controls. By using equations I and II the construction of a position assigned to weighted observations in an endometrial specimen may serve to compare the effects of drug treatment on tissue morphometry to those of the natural cycle.

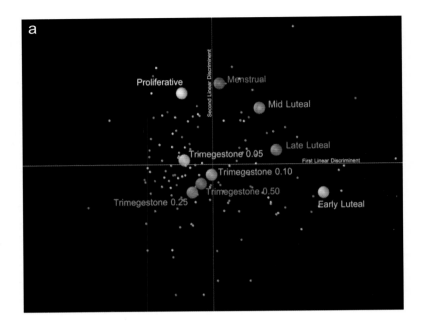

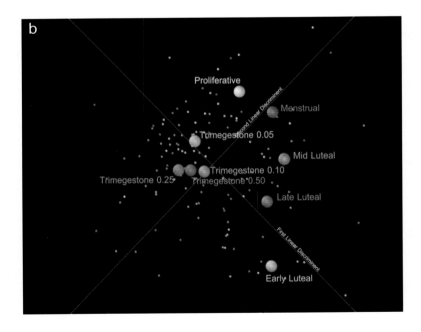

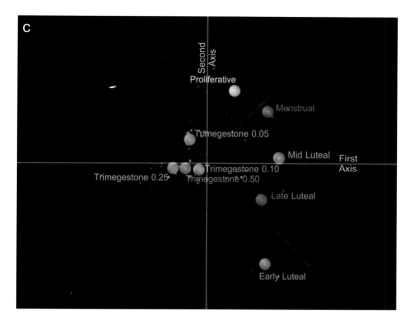

Figure 6.2. Linear discriminant analysis of 13 histologic variables. (**a**) A two-dimensional plot which preserves the relationship between group means, and maximally distinguishes between the phases of the natural cycle and the doses of trimegestone; the large circles represent the group means and smaller circles represent data from individual women. The phases of the natural cycle are shown as circles of darkening shades of red, and the doses of trimegestone as circles of darkening shades of blue; (**b**) the figure has been rotated through 45° (clockwise); (**c**) the result of using weighted values of ≥ 0.4 to construct the plot

ENDOMETRIAL SAFETY IN CLINICAL TRIALS

In drug development studies the endometrial safety profile of a given progestogen is presented at three levels:

(1) An adequate number of women, usually 300–350, are treated with the proposed regimen for 1–2 years, and the incidence of endometrial hyperplasia and carcinoma in the end-of-study biopsy is evaluated against the natural incidence in the untreated population.

(2) The induction of secretory changes in the endometrium is considered as an efficacy parameter for that progestogen. Furthermore, it is implicitly accepted as a surrogate measure for the anti-hyperplasia/carcinoma effect.

Table 6.2. Standardized weights for the rotated scales shown in Figure 6.2b. Data from Wahab M, Thompson J, Hamid B, *et al. Hum Reprod* 1999;14:2609–18

	Rotated linear discriminant functions	
Histologic parameters	1	2
% glandular area	0.92	0.84
% vascular space area	0.71	−0.81
Average glandular diameter	−0.14	−0.50
Average vascular space diameter	0.07	0.40
Stromal cell count	0.08	0.12
No. of complete glands	0.09	−0.39
No. of 'half' glands	−0.04	0.20
% gland with columnar lining	0.37	−0.28
No. of vascular spaces	−0.07	0.28
% gland with vacuoles	−0.40	0.67
% gland with secretions	0.28	−0.18
% gland with telescoping	−0.44	0.25
% gland with smooth surface	0.29	0.21

(3)   The pattern of uterine bleeding, as a result, is established within two to three treatment cycles, but it may take several years to prove the protective effect of a progestogen against endometrial neoplasia.

These biopsies are usually taken at the end of the progestogen phase of the last treatment cycle of the study. Not only do these biopsies represent a single observation point of endometrial development under the effect of a given HRT regimen, but a significant number of women may have bled by then with the consequence that a subset of these biopsies will show proliferative endometrium. Another approach has been used, where the biopsy is obtained after 8–10 days of the commencement of the administration of the progestogen in the last treatment cycle. This gives a better opportunity to demonstrate the extent of secretory transformation in a large number of treated endometria, but at the same time opens the question of how these changes compare between different treatment regimens, and how any of these changes compare to which stage of the luteal phase of the natural cycle. This is logical since synthetic progestogens are different from natural progesterone in their interaction with the progesterone, androgen and estrogen receptors. In addition, different bleeding patterns depend on factors such as dose and duration of progestogen administration. The components of endometrial tissue treated with exogenous sex steroids at any given point may keep pace to a greater or lesser extent with the respective secretory transformations of the components of the endometrium of the natural cycle, making the assignment of the phase of development largely subjective.

CONCLUSION

There is a need to devise a method whereby the changes and the degree of variability in individual components of the endometrium of the natural cycle can be evaluated and given standardized weighting for the total assessment of tissues from that phase of the cycle. Only then can one draw any comparison on the susceptibility of the particular component of the endometrium to a given progestogen. This may further our understanding of the effects of these drugs, and allow an objective approach to dealing with endometrial instability during the HRT cycle.

REFERENCES

1. Shaw ST Jr, Macaulay LK, Hohman WR. Vessel density in endometrium of women with and without intrauterine contraceptive devices: a morphometric evaluation. *Am J Obstet Gynecol* 1979;135:202–6
2. Mazur MM, Kurman RJ. *Diagnosis of Endometrial Biopsies and Curettage: a Practical Approach*. New York: Springer, 1995:8,23,234
3. Noyes RW, Hertig AT, Rock J. Dating the endometrial biopsy. *Fertil Steril* 1950;1: 3–25
4. Dallenbach-Hellweg G, Poulsen H, eds. *Atlas of Endometrial Histopathology*. New York: Springer, 1996:4,109
5. Whitehead MI, Pickar J. Variation between pathologists in the reporting of endometrial histology with combination oestrogen/progestogen therapies. *Maturitas* 1997;27(Suppl):192
6. Johannisson E. Endometrial morphology during the normal cycle and under the influence of contraceptive steroids. In D'Arcangues C, Fraser IS, Newton JR, Odlind V, eds. *Contraception and Mechanism of Endometrial Bleeding*. Cambridge: Cambridge University Press, 1990:53–80
7. Landgren BM, Johannisson E, Xing S, *et al*. A clinical pharmacological study of a new type of vaginal delivery system for levonorgestrel. *Contraception* 1985;32:581–601
8. Croxatto HD, Diaz S, Pavez M, Croxatto HB. Histopathology of the endometrium during continuous use of levonorgestrel. In Zatuchni GI, Goldsmith A, Shelton JD, Sciarra JJ, eds. *Long-acting Contraceptive Delivery Systems*. Philadelphia: Harper & Row, 1984:290–5

9. Rogers PA, Au CL, Affandi B. Endometrial microvascular density during the normal menstrual cycle and following exposure to long-term levonorgestrel. *Hum Reprod* 1993;8:1396–404

10. Song JY, Markham R, Russell P, *et al*. The effect of high-dose medium- and long-term progestogen exposure on endometrial vessels. *Hum Reprod* 1995;10:797–800

11. Sheppard BL, Bonnar J. The effects of intrauterine contraceptive devices on the ultra-structure of the endometrium in relation to bleeding complications. *Am J Obstet Gynecol* 1983;146:829–39

12. Wahab M, Thompson J, Al-Azzawi F. Effect of different cyclical sequential progestins on endometrial vascularity in postmenopausal women compared with the natural cycle: a morphometric analysis. *Hum Reprod* 2000;15:2075–81

13. Kendall BS, Ronnett BM, Isacson C, *et al*. Reproducibility of the diagnosis of endometrial hyperplasia, atypical hyperplasia, and well-differentiated carcinoma. *Am J Surg Pathol* 1998;22:1012–19

14. Johannisson E, Brosens I, Cornillie F, *et al*. Morphometric study of the human endometrium following continuous exposure to levonorgestrel released from vaginal rings during 90 days. *Contraception* 1991;43:361–74

15. Johannisson E, Landgren BM, Rohr HP, Diczfalusy E. Endometrial morphology and peripheral hormone levels in women with regular menstrual cycles. *Fertil Steril* 1987; 48:401–8

16. Ludwig H. The morphologic response of the human endometrium to long-term treatment with progestational agents. *Am J Obstet Gynecol* 1982;142:796–808

17. Casanas-Roux F, Nisolle M, Marbaix E, *et al*. Morphometric, immunohistological and three-dimensional evaluation of the endometrium of menopausal women treated by oestrogen and Crinone, a new slow-release vaginal progesterone. *Hum Reprod* 1996;11: 357–63

18. Habiba MA, Bell SC, Al-Azzawi F. Endometrial responses to hormone replacement therapy: histological features compared with those of late luteal phase endometrium. *Hum Reprod* 1998;13:1674–82

19. Wahab M, Thompson J, Hamid B, *et al*. Endometrial histomorphometry of trimegestone-based sequential hormone replacement therapy: a weighted comparison with the endo-metrium of the natural cycle. *Hum Reprod* 1999;14:2609–18

20. Wahab M, Thompson J, Al-Azzawi F. The effect of submucous fibroids on the dose-dependent modulation of uterine bleeding by trimegestone in postmenopausal women treated with hormone replacement therapy. *Br J Obstet Gynaecol* 2000;107:329–34

21. Al-Azzawi F, Wahab M, Thompson J, *et al*. Acceptability and patterns of uterine bleeding in sequential trimegestone-based hormone replacement therapy: a dose-ranging study. *Hum Reprod* 1999;14:636–41

7
Bleeding in post-reproductive years
M. Wahab and F. Al-Azzawi

INTRODUCTION

The decline in ovarian function during the fifth decade of a woman's life results in altered rates of sex steroid secretion, which are manifested by an increasing incidence of menstrual irregularities in terms of changes of rhythm, duration and severity of blood loss. In addition, such alteration in sex steroids is associated with a higher prevalence of premenstrual tension syndrome (mood swings, depression, irritability, fluid retention and mastalgia). These clinical pictures do not correlate with the measured serum levels of estradiol, progesterone or gonadotropins. Furthermore, during this time, features of estrogen deficiency that affect other systems develop insidiously, targeting particularly the collagen content of skin, bone and the supportive tissue of the reproductive organs.

ABNORMAL MENSTRUATION IN THE PERIMENOPAUSE

Abnormal menstrual bleeding after the age of 40 is common and frequently a cause for investigation. Most gynecologic literature emphasizes the need to simplify and accurately diagnose endometrial neoplasia, a condition with an increasing incidence and of potentially serious consequences. Functional disorders of the endometrium with or without the presence of polyps or submucous fibroids are much more common and the available treatment modalities are less than satisfactory. Excessive menstrual loss may lead to iron deficiency anemia and may eventually end up in hysterectomy, which is associated with significant risks of morbidity and mortality. Consequently, perimenopausal functional disorders of the endometrium demand thorough evaluation of the uterine cavity and the endometrium for the appropriate management of these disorders.

The incidence of hyperplasia is about 8%, and of atypical hyperplasia is 1.3%[1,2]. Only 3–5% of endometrial cancer cases occur in women under the age of 40[3,4]. The exclusion of a discrete pathology of the reproductive system – neoplasia, uterine fibroids, endometriosis, sex steroid treatment, the use of an intrauterine contraceptive device (IUCD), or systemic disorders such as etiologic factors for abnormal menstruation – will leave more than 80% of perimenopausal women with the diagnosis of dysfunctional uterine bleeding (DUB). Despite its low frequency, the exclusion of neoplasia is very important, but a diagnosis of benignity *per se* does not alleviate the symptoms of abnormal uterine bleeding.

Evaluation of the endometrial response

The histologic features of the endometrium in dysfunctional uterine bleeding at the premenstrual phase may either bear the signs of anovulation or show the features of luteal phase endometrium, in an estimated ratio of 1:4, respectively. Management of DUB has been achieved with the use of prostaglandin synthetase inhibitors, anti-fibrinolytic agents, combined oral contraceptive pills, and with the use of IUCDs, delivering levonorgestrel (LNG). Based on current knowledge it is prudent to differentiate between women with ovulatory and anovulatory DUB, since the supplementation of cyclical progestogens in anovulatory DUB may cure the symptoms, but it is ineffective in the management of ovulatory DUB[5]. The LNG-laden IUCD is being widely used to control DUB since the continuous delivery of LNG may induce endometrial thinness and sometimes atrophy, thus reducing the amount of blood loss. It is associated with irregular bleeding and spotting for a period of 6–9 months after the insertion of the IUCD in more than 30% of women. Furthermore, there are no data available on the long-term safety of the systemic absorption of LNG in these women.

To distinguish between ovulatory and anovulatory DUB a premenstrual endometrial sample is required, but this has logistic problems since many women with DUB have irregular periods as well, and a timely biopsy can prove difficult to obtain. The altered proportions of ovarian sex steroids produced may compromise endometrial stability leading to premature or irregular shedding, and if such hormonal influences further affect the local hemostatic mechanisms that seal the denuded blood vessels, heavy bleeding ensues. A detailed histologic assessment of premenstrual biopsy may help to elucidate features of estrogen or progesterone predominance on the endometrium[6]. The adoption of these principles may provide a better and more individualized approach to correcting dysfunctional menstrual disorders.

Detailed analysis of endometrial biopsies can be achieved using weighted variables of tissue parameters known to be modulated by estrogen or progesterone in a linear discriminant analysis model (Chapter 6)[7]. The weighted variables of histologic parameters observed in a given endometrial biopsy may be plotted against those derived from different phases of the natural cycle and the detected differences may provide a guide to the relevant hormone deficiency. A similar approach can be adopted in situations encountered with hormone replacement therapy (HRT) regimens in the absence of structural abnormalities of the endometrium.

POSTMENOPAUSAL BLEEDING

Any episode of vaginal bleeding 12 months after the last natural menstrual period (menopause) is labeled as postmenopausal bleeding. It is not normal to bleed vaginally after the menopause, unless sex steroids are being administered. Consequently, postmenopausal bleeding is potentially serious as it may be the presenting symptom of genital tract cancer and therefore necessitates a systematic approach to ensure the exclusion of malignancy.

Histologic features of the postmenopausal endometrium

The histologic features of the postmenopausal endometrium have been depicted in the literature as an inactive thin layer of luminal epithelium, with a few inactive glands lined by cuboidal or low columnar cells (Figures 7.1 and 7.2). In the majority of instances the endometrium looks atrophic or weakly proliferative. The atrophic changes and thinness of the endometrium, as a result of a lack of estrogen, may expose the endometrial capillaries and enhance their fragility; consequently they bleed. However, many such cases are investigated some time after the event, and whether a different histologic picture, resulting from a transient increase in estrogenic stimulus of the endometrium, had prevailed at the time of the bleeding episode remains speculative. In the absence of discrete pathology, the endometrium procured from women presenting with postmenopausal bleeding expresses the estrogen and progesterone receptors in a manner comparable to that of premenopausal samples, despite the fact that these women had no detectable serum estradiol levels[8]. These findings suggest that even the seemingly atrophic endometrium is an active tissue that can be made responsive to an increase in endogenous estrone as, for example, in obesity or following the administration of exogenous sex steroids.

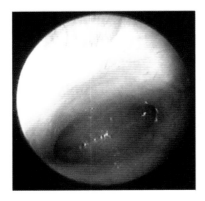 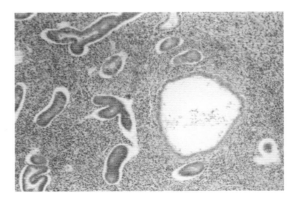

Figure 7.1. Hysteroscopic view of atrophic endometrium in a post-menopausal woman

Figure 7.2. Hematoxylin and eosin (H&E)-stained atrophic endometrium in a postmenopausal woman, original magnification × 200

Postmenopausal bleeding and associated pathology

Malignant disease of the uterine corpus, cervix and occasionally ovarian neoplasia may present as postmenopausal bleeding. The significance of postmenopausal bleeding as a 'presenting symptom' was illustrated by Gredmark and colleagues[9], who reported endometrial hyperplasia (10%), adenocarcinoma (8%), ovarian tumor (1.8%) and cervical cancer (1.3%) among 457 cases managed in one county in Sweden over 18 months. Rarely, cancer of the vagina or of the vulva is the underlying pathology. Non-genital bleeding such as hematuria or rectal bleeding is sometimes confused with vaginal bleeding, especially in the elderly. Benign uterine polyps, adenomatous or fibromyomatous, may present in this way, and potential focal neoplastic changes have to be considered. Therefore for a full diagnosis it is necessary to view the endometrial cavity by hysteroscopy and obtain an adequate biopsy for histologic assessment[10]. Other benign causes of postmenopausal bleeding are listed in Table 7.1. The most common histologic finding in women presenting with postmenopausal bleeding is, nevertheless, atrophic endometrium.

Endometrial polyps

Endometrial polyps (Figures 7.3 and 7.4) are localized outgrowths of endometrial tissue covered by epithelium which contain a variable amount of glands, stroma and blood vessels. They are encountered most commonly during the fifth decade of life. In premenopausal women they may present clinically as intermenstrual bleeding or as heavy periods, or sometimes as excessive vaginal discharge.

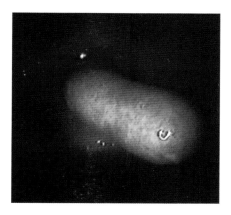

Figure 7.3. Hysteroscopic view of fibroid polyp

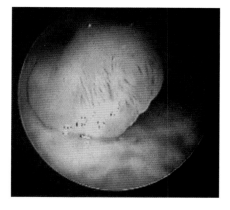

Figure 7.4. Hysteroscopic view showing fleshy polyp on the right lateral uterine wall

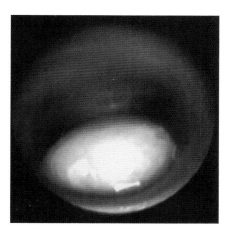

Figure 7.5. Hysteroscopic view of submucous fibroid in the posterior uterine wall

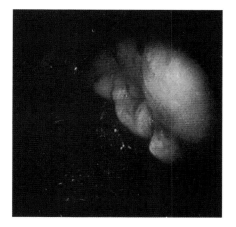

Figure 7.6. Hysteroscopic view of polypoid endometrium adjacent to submucous fibroid

Table 7.1. Benign causes of postmenopausal bleeding

Atrophic vaginitis

Cervical and endometrial polyps

Submucous fibroids

Benign ovarian neoplasms, as they may stimulate steroidogenesis in the adjacent normal ovarian stroma, or the rare estrogen-producing ovarian tumors

Use of estrogenic medications, particularly estrogen-containing vaginal creams

Endometrial polyps vary in size from 1 mm to a large fleshy mass that may protrude through the cervix. They can be broad-based and sessile, or attached to the endometrium by a slender stalk. They are usually solitary, but multiple polyps can be found as well. The glandular element of a polyp is characteristically out of phase with the rest of endometrial development, and secretory changes in these glands are seldom found. Occasionally hyperplasia or early carcinoma may develop exclusively in the polyp. There are indications of an increased incidence of endometrial hyperplasia and carcinoma in women found to have endometrial polyps[11], but this may be due to the increased propensity of such endometria to develop neoplasia rather than an inherent feature of the polyps. In a prospective cohort study involving 248 women who underwent outpatient hysteroscopy and endometrial biopsy, 62 had endometrial polyps and were compared with 186 endometrial samples which did not have polyps, taken as control. The incidence of hyperplasia in polyps was 11.3% compared to 4.3% in control samples, while the incidence of carcinoma was identical in both groups at 3.2%[12].

Removal of the polyp with endometrial curettage may be all that is required, but a confirmatory hysteroscopy is necessary, since these polyps may be so pliable that they are missed by the curettage. Where hyperplastic changes are found localized to the polyp in premenopausal women, then polypectomy with curettage may be adequate. However in postmenopausal women hysterectomy will be the appropriate choice if atypia is also present.

The role of submucous fibroids (myoma)

The presence of submucous fibroids (Figures 7.5 and 7.6) has been linked to the development of abnormal uterine bleeding. We have documented a twofold increase in the risk of having submucous fibroids in premenopausal women who presented with heavy and irregular menses, and a threefold increase for the presence of these fibroids in postmenopausal women who presented with heavy and irregular bleeding on HRT, compared to asymptomatic controls[13]. The presence of submucous fibroids has also been associated with a higher incidence of intermenstrual bleeding (IMB) in postmenopausal women on HRT[14].

The identification of polyps and submucous fibroids may help to predict the woman's response to sex steroid therapy[15], and aids the planning of local surgical management if this is deemed necessary[16]. Furthermore, two studies have shown that 87% of postmenopausal women with heavy and unscheduled bleeding on HRT improved and experienced regular bleeding on HRT when these submucous fibroids were removed by hysteroscopic surgery[17,18]. The result of this intervention, however, was less successful in premenopausal women, which adds further evidence that abnormal uterine bleeding in the presence of submucous fibroids in this group of women forms only part of the abnormal hormonal response of the endometrium. In women who present with spontaneous postmenopausal bleeding the presence of submucous fibroids or polyps was not found more often than in controls[13].

It has long been recognized that the development of the endometrium overlying the submucous fibroids is less advanced and shows a mixed picture of proliferative, secretory and poorly developed patches compared to the rest of the adjacent endometrium[19,20]. Whether such endometrial defects are due to the altered pattern of the vasculature which supplies these fibroids, or due to paracrine factors induced as a result of the development of the fibroids themselves, is not known.

ENDOMETRIAL NEOPLASIA

Incidence

Endometrial cancer has one of the highest survival rates of all cancer types and 74% of uterine cancer cases are diagnosed at a localized stage; a greater majority of women under the age of 50 have their cancer diagnosed at an early stage[21]. The incidence of endometrial carcinoma varies with race and geographic location. Adjusted for age, the rate of endometrial cancer in the USA is reported to be from 17.6 to 22.2 per 100 000 in white women and 10.4 for Afro-Caribbean women, while that among Chinese women is 10–15 times lower (Table 7.2)[22].

Risk factors

Pre-existing hyperplasia
Hyperplasia – simple or complex – is a histologic description which refers to the excessive formation of tissue owing to an increase in the number of cells; the presence of atypia divides these two categories into further subgroups. The significance of this classification lies in the rate of progression to endometrial carcinoma. Only 2% of patients with simple hyperplasia without atypia will progress to carcinoma within 7 years, but the rate is ten times higher for those with complex atypical hyperplasia[23]. What is not certain is the precise time frame required for the progression of a particular hyperplastic state to carcinoma, but the reported intervals in the literature range between 4 and 10 years[24,25].

Table 7.2. Age-adjusted incidence of endometrial cancer in different races and geographic locations. Adapted from Parkin DM. *Rev Epidemiol Sante Publique* 1992; 40:410–24[22]

Country or ethnicity	Incidence/100 000 women
White (USA)	17.6–22.2
Afro-Caribbean (USA)	10.4
Maori (New Zealand)	16.4
France	14.8
England and Wales	8.1
India	1.6–2.3
China	1.3–2.9
Japan	3.2
Japanese living in USA	12

Oral contraceptive pill

The combined oral contraceptive pill (COC) has consistently been shown to reduce the incidence of endometrial cancer by about 50%, while sequential oral contraceptives are found to increase the risk by twofold at least[26,27]. The longer is the duration of use of the COC, the better is the protection against endometrial cancer; a decrease in the risk of the disease of 23% after 1 year of use progresses to a 70% decrease among women who use COCs for 12 years[28]. The effect of COCs on reducing the risk of endometrial cancer is independent of age at first use[28,29] or of the dose or potency of the progestin among long-term users[30]. The protective effect of COCs may last for several years after discontinuation[28,31,32]. Whether such protective effects may still be conferred upon unopposed estrogen users in the postmenopause is not known[33,34].

Parity

The nulliparous woman has a threefold increase in the risk of endometrial cancer compared to parous women, an effect which appears to be related to the number of full-term pregnancies[35,36]. Furthermore, infertility as a result of anovulation or polycystic ovary syndrome has been identified as a high-risk factor for the development of endometrial cancer[35,37].

Body weight

Obesity induces a variety of alterations in reproductive function, including irregularity of menstrual cycles and reduction in the frequency of ovulation[38].

Obesity in general is associated with a threefold increase in the risk of endometrial cancer[39]. Even among Chinese women, where the incidences of obesity and of endometrial cancer are low, general obesity and fat deposits over the trunk are associated with a doubling of the risk[40]. Central obesity – independent of body mass index – was found in some studies not to be associated with an increased risk[39,40], but others showed it to increase the risk in a linear fashion[41]. Whether the associated hyperinsulinemia and increased levels of insulin-like growth factor-I (IGF-I) may contribute to this heightened risk is not known.

Diabetes mellitus
Postmenopausal women with type II diabetes mellitus have an increased estrogen level[42] and a twofold increase in the risk of endometrial cancer[36]. It is not known whether specific features of the diabetic status or the consequences of the mitogenic effect of hyperinsulinemia and raised IGF-I level are responsible for this heightened risk.

Menstrual characteristics
Early menarche, particularly under the age of 12, and, more significantly, late menopause – after the age of 55 – are cited as factors of increased risk for the development of endometrial cancer[35,36]. This may be attributed to the high number of anovulatory cycles to which the endometrium has been exposed. Similarly elevated risks are described in women with menstrual irregularities such as heavy periods, long cycles and amenorrhea and in those experiencing premenstrual fluid retention[36,43]. These findings may reflect the abnormal endocrine milieu associated with these disorders.

Lifestyle
A number of case–control studies have suggested that lifestyle factors might be implicated in modifying the risks for endometrial cancer; however, the data are inconclusive. High total calorie consumption and high caloric intake from animal and vegetable fats are moderate risks for this cancer, while high consumption of fruit, vegetables, bread and cereals is associated with lower risks[27,44,45]. An evaluation of the association of physical activity, weight and weight change, fruit, vegetables and alcohol consumption, socio-economic status, parity, or the presence of diabetes mellitus with the risk of endometrial cancer was reported in a cohort study. There was no clear pattern of risk over levels of alcohol or fruit and vegetable intake, although the data suggest an increased risk with very low fruit and vegetable intake, while increasing physical activity markedly decreased the risk of endometrial cancer[46]. Cigarette smoking has been shown consistently to reduce the risk of this

cancer[47–50]. This may be related to the induction of the 2-hydroxylase enzyme, which inactivates the majority of circulating estrogens into catechol estrogens, or it may be due to the induction of early menopause as a result of a direct toxic effect of tobacco smoking on the reserve of oocytes.

HORMONAL TREATMENT AND ENDOMETRIAL CANCER

HRT use and endometrial cancer

Chronic unopposed estrogen administration induces a proliferative endometrium, which progresses to a well-differentiated endometrial adenocarcinoma in a significant number of women. Such a progress is thought to pass through several intermediary stages of proliferation of increasing complexity, collectively termed 'endometrial hyperplasia'. The duration of use of unopposed estrogen in postmenopausal women remains the strongest predictor for the development of endometrial cancer. The relative risk increases exponentially from 1.4 (95% confidence interval (CI), 1.0–1.8) for less than 1 year of use, to 9.5 (95% CI, 7.4–12.3) among users for 10 years or more[51].

The effect of unopposed estrogen use on the risk of endometrial cancer is also directly related to the dose of estrogen[36,51,52] although a consistent dose–response relationship is lacking. Cessation of therapy results in a rapid decline of the risk within about 2 years but may remain higher than in the non-user population for up to 10–15 years[51,53]. The cyclical addition of progestogen for 10–14 days each month to continuously administered estrogen has been shown to confer a reduction in the risk of endometrial hyperplasia and cancer[30,54,55]. However, this addition of a progestogen does not eliminate the increased risk: 1.9 (95% CI, 0.9–3.8) compared to 6.5 (95% CI, 3.1–13.3) for the unopposed estrogen user[34,52]. Indeed, Weiderpass and colleagues showed that sequential regimens, with the progestogen being administered for fewer than 16 days in a 28-day treatment cycle, were associated with an increased risk of endometrial cancer with an odds ratio (OR) of 2.9 (95% CI, 1.8–4.6) for 5 or more years of use[32]. In the same article users of continuous combined HRT (ccHRT) were reported as enjoying significant protection against endometrial hyperplasia and cancer, OR 0.2 (95% CI, 0.1–1.8) for 5 or more years of use. The increased risk of endometrial cancer was dependent on the type and duration (days per treatment cycle) of the progestogen used. For example, 19-nortestosterone derivatives conferred higher protection compared to the progesterone-derived progestins.

The occurrence of an unscheduled or abnormal bleeding pattern in postmeno-pausal women using HRT – continuous combined or a sequential regimen – should be considered as postmenopausal bleeding and managed as such. In women using ccHRT the occurrence of irregular bleeding during the first 3 months of treatment is quite common. A full investigation will be required if such bleeding lasts for more than 6 months and investigation may be indicated earlier in women with higher risks of developing endometrial neoplasia such as in cases of obesity, diabetes mellitus, nulliparity[56] or a family history of colonic carcinoma[57]. In one population-based study the incidence of adenomatous and atypical hyperplasia was estimated at 44 per 100 000 per year and overall obesity, rather than specific regional distribution of fat, was characteristic of these women[58]. Despite the identification of risk factors, investigation of the endometrium cannot safely be withheld from women who do not have these risks[56].

Poor compliance with HRT

Irregular use of HRT regimens is an important issue that deserves thorough con-sideration in the clinical assessment of women presenting with heavy or unscheduled bleeding, since missing tablets, for example, may alter the bio-availability of sex steroid, render the endometrium unstable and cause bleeding. Where progestogenic adverse effects are experienced, women try to stop using part or the whole of the progestogen phase of the HRT regimen, to avoid these symptoms. It is estimated that about 30% of women who are prescribed sequential combined HRT regimens stop taking the progestogen component owing to symp-toms of fluid retention, bloatedness, mastalgia and mood swings; consequently, the endometrial changes will be similar to those with unopposed estrogen. In the Postmenopausal Estrogen/Progestin Interventions (PEPI) trial[59], 62.5% of women with an intact uterus who used unopposed estrogen for 3 years developed abnormal bleeding or had an abnormal Papanicolaou test which necessitated further investigation. Eighty per cent of unopposed estrogen users had endometrial abnormalities, of which 80.5% were simple hyperplasia, 18.8% atypical hyperplasia, and 0.7% were endometrial carcinoma.

TAMOXIFEN

Tamoxifen, a non-steroidal anti-estrogen, is currently the endocrine therapy of choice for all stages of breast cancer, in which it has been shown to improve both the disease-free interval and the survival rates of postmenopausal women diag-nosed with this cancer. As adjuvant therapy it has been shown that more than

2 years of tamoxifen treatment is more effective than a shorter course. In breast tissue it is believed to act by competitive inhibition at the estrogen receptor, preventing full activation of the estrogen-responsive genes. However, the degree of inhibition or activation of estrogen receptor genes varies between different tissue types.

There is an increased incidence of endometrial polyps in tamoxifen users compared to that in the general population (8–36% versus 0–10%, respectively)[60–63]. These polyps may be the source of uterine bleeding but they are asymptomatic in the main. Polyps associated with tamoxifen treatment are characterized by dilated cystic glands, metaplastic epithelial changes and focal stromal condensation around the glands[64], with extensive stromal fibrosis (Figures 7.7 and 7.8). Stromal fibrosis may account for the difficulty in sampling the endometrium under the effect of tamoxifen. Endometrial hyperplasia occurs at a higher rate in tamoxifen-treated women: 2–20% versus 0–10% in the general population, respectively[63,65–71]. The histologic picture is classified similarly to that of other endometrial hyperplasias not associated with tamoxifen treatment, i.e. simple or complex hyperplasia with or without atypia (see above). In tamoxifen-treated women the relative risk of endometrial carcinoma is increased by 1.3–7.5-fold, and such risk is directly related to the dose and duration of use[63,68,70,72–75]; more evidence for this finding was contained in a recent report of a case–control study from The Netherlands[76]. However, despite rigorous follow-up in clinical trials, the Dutch report showed a more advanced International Federation of Gynecologists and Obstetricians (FIGO) staging (III and IV) in about one-fifth of tamoxifen users who developed endometrial carcinoma, with a high incidence of mixed mesodermal tumors and

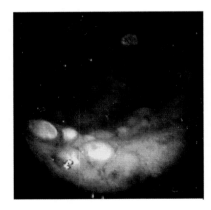

Figure 7.7. Hysteroscopic view of cystic endometrium in postmenopausal woman treated with tamoxifen

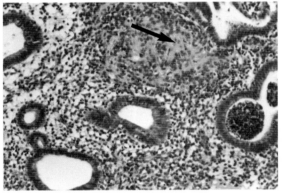

Figure 7.8. Hematoxylin and eosin (H&E) stain of endometrium in a tamoxifen-treated woman (original magnification × 200). Arrow, stromal fibrosis

sarcomas: 5.4%, versus 2.9% in the untreated controls. The high prevalence of p53-positive endometrial tumors in this study is suggestive of an increasing likelihood of a poor prognosis.

In another trial hysteroscopy and endometrial biopsy obtained prior to commencement of tamoxifen treatment in breast cancer patients identified endometrial polyps in about 17% of asymptomatic women. Over a period of 3 years of follow-up women with initially benign lesions of the uterus had a statistically significantly higher chance of developing atypical lesions, including carcinoma *in situ*[77]. In breast cancer prevention trials the relative risk for endometrial cancer associated with tamoxifen administration is estimated at about 2.5-fold[78]. Given the low incidence of endometrial cancer in the general population, the cost–benefit analysis remains in favor of the administration of tamoxifen, be that as an adjuvant chemotherapy or as a chemopreventive agent in high-risk groups.

Overview of management of tamoxifen-related disorders

The increased incidence of endometrial pathology may justify all women with breast cancer who are being treated with tamoxifen undergoing an annual gynecologic examination, including a rectovaginal examination and a cervical smear for cytologic assessment. However, there is a diversity of opinion regarding the timing and the extent of investigation in the asymptomatic patient. Women who develop vaginal bleeding, regardless of its severity or duration, should be fully evaluated clinically, the uterus and appendages being assessed by transvaginal ultrasound scan and the endometrial cavity being examined by hysteroscopy. It is imperative that an adequate endometrial biopsy are obtained; in these patients a sample suitable for histologic diagnosis was obtained in only 85% of patients even with the use of a sharp curette, following office hysteroscopy[79]. Cohen and colleagues[80] compared the incidence of endometrial pathology in 14 symptomatic women treated with tamoxifen with that in 224 asymptomatic tamoxifen-treated women. In view of the low incidence of malignancy in the asymptomatic women, full surveillance was not recommended and full investigation with hysteroscopy and endometrial biopsy was restricted to those with endometrial thickness in excess of 7 mm, as measured by transvaginal ultrasound. However, the finding of endometrial carcinoma in a tamoxifen-treated woman with an endometrial thickness of 3 mm highlights the falsely reassuring concept of cut-off points in endometrial thickness[63].

Should atypical hyperplasia develop, consideration should be given to discontinuing tamoxifen and instigating high-dose progestogen therapy. In the opinion of the author, hysterectomy may be a more prudent option in order to allow the continuation of tamoxifen treatment, particularly if endometrial disease is confirmed within 2 years of the diagnosis of breast cancer. The treatment of choice for those women who develop endometrial cancer is hysterectomy with removal of both ovaries. An alternative option may be offered to women with simple or complex hyperplasia without atypia by fitting them with an LNG-laden IUCD (Mirena® coil, Schering, UK) to be followed by endometrial biopsy 6–12 months later. In asymptomatic women treated with tamoxifen for 2 or more years, the use of the Mirena coil resulted in secretory transformation of the endometrium after 1 year of use in 40 cases out of 47[81]. This treatment approach is, therefore, encouraging, but it awaits further studies on its long-term safety, especially in the light of the reported detrimental effect of progestogens on breast cancer risk[82].

Ideally, women starting tamoxifen treatment should undergo pretreatment screening with a transvaginal ultrasound, but this is adequate only if the endometrial echo is thin and uniform. Otherwise, outpatient hysteroscopy is performed. For asymptomatic women further assessment will be required annually after 2–3 years from the commencement of treatment.

CONCLUSION

An abnormal bleeding pattern in the late reproductive and postmenopausal years is common and necessitates investigation. In the perimenopausal years functional disorders of the endometrium are more common than endometrial hyperplasia and carcinoma. It is prudent to differentiate between ovulatory and non-ovulatory DUB since the treatment options are different. Postmenopausal bleeding is more serious, and malignant diseases, especially of the uterus and cervix, have to be excluded, although in the majority of instances only atrophic endometrium is identified. The increasing number of postmenopausal women being treated with HRT is associated with an increase in the number of women presenting with unscheduled or abnormal bleeding. The identification of structural abnormalities affecting the uterine cavity and their subsequent removal may enhance the acceptability of the long-term continuation of HRT.

REFERENCES

1. Sherman AI. Precursors of endometrial cancer. *Isr J Med Sci* 1978;14:370–8
2. Wentz WB. Progestin therapy in endometrial hyperplasia. *Gynecol Oncol* 1974;2:362–7

3. Crissman JD, Azoury RS, Barnes AE, Schellhas HF. Endometrial carcinoma in women 40 years of age or younger. *Obstet Gynecol* 1981;57:699–704

4. Gallup DG, Stock RJ. Adenocarcinoma of the endometrium in women 40 years of age or younger. *Obstet Gynecol* 1984;64:417–20

5. Cameron IT, Leask R, Kelly RW, Baird DT. The effects of danazol, mefenamic acid, norethisterone and a progesterone-impregnated coil on endometrial prostaglandin concentrations in women with menorrhagia. *Prostaglandins* 1987;34:99–110

6. Good RG, Moyer DL. Estrogen–progesterone relationships in the development of secretory endometrium. *Fertil Steril* 1968;19:37–49

7. Wahab M, Thompson J, Hamid B, *et al.* Endometrial histomorphometry of trimegestone-based sequential hormone replacement therapy: a weighted comparison with the endometrium of the natural cycle. *Hum Reprod* 1999;14:2609–18

8. Gorodeski GI, Bahary CM. Expression of estradiol and progesterone receptors by histologically normal endometria of women with postmenopausal bleeding. *J Endocrinol Invest* 1991;14:537–42

9. Gredmark T, Kvint S, Havel G, Mattsson LA. Histopathological findings in women with postmenopausal bleeding. *Br J Obstet Gynaecol* 1995;102:133–6

10. Orvieto R, Bar-Hava I, Dicker D, *et al.* Endometrial polyps during menopause: characterization and significance. *Acta Obstet Gynecol Scand* 1999;78:883–6

11. Armenia CS. Sequential relationship between endometrial polyps and carcinoma of the endometrium. *Obstet Gynecol* 1967;30:524–9

12. Bakour SH, Khan KS, Gupta JK. The risk of premalignant and malignant pathology in endometrial polyps. *Acta Obstet Gynecol Scand* 2000;79:317–20

13. Akkad AA, Habiba MA, Ismail N, *et al.* Abnormal uterine bleeding on hormone replacement: the importance of intrauterine structural abnormalities. *Obstet Gynecol* 1995;86:330–4

14. Wahab M, Thompson J, Al-Azzawi F. The effect of submucous fibroids on the dose-dependent modulation of uterine bleeding by trimegestone in postmenopausal women treated with hormone replacement therapy. *Br J Obstet Gynaecol* 2000;107:329–34

15. Downes E, Al-Azzawi F. The predictive value of outpatient hysteroscopy in a menopause clinic – a prospective study of 254 patients. *Br J Obstet Gynaecol* 1993;100:1148–9

16. Neuwirth RS. Hysteroscopic submucous myomectomy. *Obstet Gynecol Clin North Am* 1995;22:541–58

17. Al-Azzawi F. Prediction of successful outcome following hysteroscopic laser myomectomy in women with heavy and unscheduled bleeding. *Climacteric* 1999;2(Suppl):289

18. Cravello L, de Montgolfier R, D'Ercole C, *et al.* Hysteroscopic surgery in post-menopausal women. *Acta Obstet Gynecol Scand* 1996;75:563–6

19. Mazur MM, Kurman RJ. *Diagnosis of Endometrial Biopsies and Curettage: a Practical Approach.* New York: Springer, 1995;8,23,234

20. Dallenbach-Hellweg G, Poulsen H, eds. *Atlas of Endometrial Histopathology.* New York: Springer, 1996:105–9

21. Miller BA, Ries LAG, Hankey BF, eds. *SEER Cancer Statistics Review: 1973–1990.* Bethesda, MD: United States Department of Health and Human Services, 1993

22. Parkin DM. Studies of cancer in migrant populations: methods and interpretation. *Rev Epidemiol Sante Publique* 1992;40:410–24

23. Kurman RJ, Zaino RJ, Norris HJ. Endometrial carcinoma. In Kurman RJ, ed. *Blaustein's Pathology of the Female Genital Tract,* volume 4. New York: Springer, 1994:439–86

24. Pettersson B, Adami HO, Lindgren A, Hesselius I. Endometrial polyps and hyperplasia as risk factors for endometrial carcinoma. A case–control study of curettage specimens. *Acta Obstet Gynecol Scand* 1985;64:653–9

25. Kurman RJ, Kaminski PF, Norris HJ. The behavior of endometrial hyperplasia. A long-term study of 'untreated' hyperplasia in 170 patients. *Cancer* 1985;56:403–12

26. Jick SS. Combined estrogen and progesterone use and endometrial cancer [Letter]. *Epidemiology* 1993;4:384

27. Levi F, Franceschi S, Negri E, La Vecchia C. Dietary factors and the risk of endometrial cancer. *Cancer* 1993;71:3575–81

28. Schlesselman JJ. Oral contraceptives and neoplasia of the uterine corpus. *Contraception* 1991;43:557–79

29. Jick SS, Walker AM, Jick H. Oral contraceptives and endometrial cancer. *Obstet Gynecol* 1993;82:931–5

30. Voigt LF, Weiss NS, Chu J, *et al.* Progestagen supplementation of exogenous oestrogens and risk of endometrial cancer. *Lancet* 1991;338:274–7

31. van Leeuwen FE, Rookus MA. The role of exogenous hormones in the epidemiology of breast, ovarian and endometrial cancer. *Eur J Cancer Clin Oncol* 1989;25:1961–72

32. Weiderpass E, Adami HO, Baron JA, *et al.* Risk of endometrial cancer following estrogen replacement with and without progestins. *J Natl Cancer Inst* 1999;91:1131–7

33. Rubin GL, Peterson HB, Lee NC, *et al.* Estrogen replacement therapy and the risk of endometrial cancer: remaining controversies. *Am J Obstet Gynecol* 1990;162:148–54

34. Brinton LA, Hoover RN. Estrogen replacement therapy and endometrial cancer risk: unresolved issues. The Endometrial Cancer Collaborative Group. *Obstet Gynecol* 1993; 81:265–71

35. Parazzini F, La Vecchia C, Negri E, *et al.* Reproductive factors and risk of endometrial cancer. *Am J Obstet Gynecol* 1991;164:522–7

36. Brinton LA, Berman ML, Mortel R, *et al.* Reproductive, menstrual, and medical risk factors for endometrial cancer: results from a case-control study. *Am J Obstet Gynecol* 1992;167:1317–25

37. Escobedo LG, Lee NC, Peterson HB, Wingo PA. Infertility-associated endometrial cancer risk may be limited to specific subgroups of infertile women. *Obstet Gynecol* 1991;77:124–8

38. Bray GA. Obesity and reproduction. *Hum Reprod* 1997;12:26–32

39. Sherman ME, Sturgeon S, Brinton LA, *et al.* Risk factors and hormone levels in patients with serous and endometrioid uterine carcinomas. *Mod Pathol* 1997;10:963–8

40. Shu XO, Brinton LA, Zheng W, *et al.* Relation of obesity and body fat distribution to endometrial cancer in Shanghai, China. *Cancer Res* 1992;52:3865–70

41. Swanson CA, Potischman N, Wilbanks GD, *et al.* Relation of endometrial cancer risk to past and contemporary body size and body fat distribution. *Cancer Epidemiol Biomarkers Prev* 1993;2:321–7

42. Quinn MA, Ruffe H, Brown JB, Ennis G. Circulating gonadotrophins and urinary oestrogens in postmenopausal diabetic women. *Aust N Z J Obstet Gynaecol* 1981;21:234–6

43. Parazzini F, La Vecchia C, Bocciolone I, Franceschi S. The epidemiology of endometrial cancer. *Gynecol Oncol* 1991;41:1–16

44. La Vecchia C, Negri E, Franceschi S, Levi F. An epidemiological study of endometrial cancer, nutrition and health. *Eur J Cancer Prev* 1997;6:171–4

45. Cline JM, Hughes CL Jr. Phytochemicals for the prevention of breast and endometrial cancer. *Cancer Treat Res* 1998;94:107–34

46. Terry P, Baron JA, Weiderpass E, *et al.* Lifestyle and endometrial cancer risk: a cohort study from the Swedish Twin Registry. *Int J Cancer* 1999;82:38–42

47. Baron JA. Beneficial effects of nicotine and cigarette smoking: the real, the possible and the spurious. *Br Med Bull* 1996;52:58–73

48. Lesko SM, Rosenberg L, Kaufman DW, *et al.* Cigarette smoking and the risk of endometrial cancer. *N Engl J Med* 1985;313:593–6

49. Stockwell HG, Lyman GH. Cigarette smoking and the risk of female reproductive cancer. *Am J Obstet Gynecol* 1987;157:35–40

50. Brinton LA, Barrett RJ, Berman ML, *et al.* Cigarette smoking and the risk of endometrial cancer. *Am J Epidemiol* 1993;137:281–91

51. Grady D, Gebretsadik T, Kerlikowske K, *et al.* Hormone replacement therapy and endometrial cancer risk: a meta-analysis. *Obstet Gynecol* 1995;85:304–13

52. Jick SS, Walker AM, Jick H. Estrogens, progesterone, and endometrial cancer. *Epidemiology* 1993;4:20–4

53. Finkle WD, Greenland S, Miettinen OS, Ziel HK. Endometrial cancer risk after discontinuing use of unopposed conjugated estrogens (California, United States). *Cancer Causes Control* 1995;6:99–102

54. Persson I. Risk of endometrial cancer after treatment with oestrogens alone or in conjunction with progestogens; results of a prospective study. *Br Med J* 1989;298:147–51

55. Woodruff JD, Pickar JH. Incidence of endometrial hyperplasia in postmenopausal women taking conjugated estrogens (Premarin) with medroxyprogesterone acetate or conjugated estrogens alone. The Menopause Study Group. *Am J Obstet Gynecol* 1994; 170:1213–23

56. Weber AM, Belinson JL, Piedmonte MR. Risk factors for endometrial hyperplasia and cancer among women with abnormal bleeding. *Obstet Gynecol* 1999;93:594–8

57. Farquhar CM, Lethaby A, Sowter M, *et al.* An evaluation of risk factors for endometrial hyperplasia in premenopausal women with abnormal menstrual bleeding. *Am J Obstet Gynecol* 1999;181:525–9

58. Gredmark T, Kvint S, Havel G, Mattsson L. Adipose tissue distribution in postmenopausal women with adenomatous hyperplasia of the endometrium. *Gynecol Oncol* 1999;72:138–42

59. The Writing Group for the PEPI Trial. Effects of hormone replacement therapy on endometrial histology in postmenopausal women. The Postmenopausal Estrogen/Progestin Interventions (PEPI) Trial. *J Am Med Assoc* 1996;275:370–5

60. Hulka CA, Hall DA. Endometrial abnormalities associated with tamoxifen therapy for breast cancer: sonographic and pathologic correlation. *Am J Roentgenol* 1993;160:809–12

61. Jaeger BM, Brumbach K. Tamoxifen induced endometrial abnormalities: evaluation by saline infusion sonohysterography. *Md Med J* 1997;46:433–5

62. Ramondetta LM, Sherwood JB, Dunton CJ, Palazzo JP. Endometrial cancer in polyps associated with tamoxifen use. *Am J Obstet Gynecol* 1999;180:340–1

63. Seoud M, Shemseddine A, Khalil A, *et al.* Tamoxifen and endometrial pathologies: a prospective study. *Gynecol Oncol* 1999;75:15–19

64. Corley D, Rowe J, Curtis MT, *et al.* Postmenopausal bleeding from unusual endometrial polyps in women on chronic tamoxifen therapy. *Obstet Gynecol* 1992;79:111–16

65. Barakat RR. Benign and hyperplastic endometrial changes associated with tamoxifen use. *Oncology (Huntingt)* 1997;11:35–7

66. Fotiou S, Tserkezoglou A, Hadjieleftheriou G, *et al.* Tamoxifen associated uterine pathology in breast cancer patients with abnormal bleeding. *Anticancer Res* 1998;18:625–9

67. Ozsener S, Ozaran A, Itil I, Dikmen Y. Endometrial pathology of 104 postmenopausal breast cancer patients treated with tamoxifen. *Eur J Gynaecol Oncol* 1998;19:580–3

68. Schlesinger C, Kamoi S, Ascher SM, *et al.* Endometrial polyps: a comparison study of patients receiving tamoxifen with two control groups. *Int J Gynecol Pathol* 1998;17:302–11

69. Berliere M, Galant C, Donnez J. The potential oncogenic effect of tamoxifen on the endometrium. *Hum Reprod* 1999;14:1381–3

70. Cohen I, Azaria R, Aviram R, *et al.* Postmenopausal endometrial pathologies with tamoxifen treatment: comparison between hysteroscopic and hysterectomy findings. *Gynecol Obstet Invest* 1999;48:187–92

71. Kennedy MM, Baigrie CF, Manek S. Tamoxifen and the endometrium: review of 102 cases and comparison with HRT-related and non-HRT-related endometrial pathology. *Int J Gynecol Pathol* 1999;18:130–7

72. De Muylder X, Neven P, De Somer M, *et al.* Endometrial lesions in patients undergoing tamoxifen therapy. *Int J Gynaecol Obstet* 1991;36:127–30

73. Friedl A, Jordan VC. What do we know and what don't we know about tamoxifen in the human uterus. *Breast Cancer Res Treat* 1994;31:27–39

74. Ismail SM. Pathology of endometrium treated with tamoxifen. *J Clin Pathol* 1994;47: 827–33

75. Stearns V, Gelmann EP. Does tamoxifen cause cancer in humans? *J Clin Oncol* 1998;16: 779–92

76. Bergman L, Beelen ML, Gallee MP, *et al.* Risk and prognosis of endometrial cancer after tamoxifen for breast cancer. Comprehensive Cancer Centres' ALERT Group. Assessment of liver and endometrial cancer risk following tamoxifen. *Lancet* 2000;356:881–7

77. Berliere M, Charles A, Galant C, Donnez J. Uterine side effects of tamoxifen: a need for systemic pretreatment screening. *Obstet Gynecol* 1998;91:40–4

78. Fisher B, Costantino JP, Wickerham DL, *et al.* Tamoxifen for prevention of breast cancer: report of the National Surgical Adjuvant Breast and Bowel Project P-1 Study. *J Natl Cancer Inst* 1998;90:1371–88

79. Gardner FJE, Konje JC, Abrams K, *et al.* Uterine surveillance of asymptomatic postmenopausal women taking tamoxifen. *Climacteric* 1998;1:180–7

80. Cohen I, Perel E, Tepper R, *et al.* Dose-dependent effect of tamoxifen therapy on endometrial pathologies in postmenopausal breast cancer patients. *Breast Cancer Res Treat* 1999;53:255–62

81. Gardner FJ, Konje JC, Abrams KR, *et al.* Endometrial protection from tamoxifen-stimulated changes by a levonorgestrel-releasing intrauterine system: a randomised controlled trial. *Lancet* 2000;356:1711–17

82. Schairer C, Lubin J, Troisi R, *et al.* Menopausal estrogen and estrogen–progestin replacement therapy and breast cancer risk. *J Am Med Assoc* 2000;283:485–91

8
Evaluation of diagnostic techniques
F. Al-Azzawi and M. Wahab

INTRODUCTION

One of the fundamental principles in clinical practice is the achievement of an accurate diagnosis with minimal inconvenience to the patient. The value of a given diagnostic procedure is measured by the specificity and sensitivity of the test, along with the estimated positive and negative predictive values.

TERMINOLOGY

The sensitivity of a test is the proportion of positives that are correctly identified by it; the specificity is the proportion of negatives that are correctly identified; the positive predictive value is the proportion of patients with positive test results who are correctly diagnosed; and the negative predictive value is the proportion of patients with negative test results who are correctly diagnosed (Table 8.1).

The sensitivity, specificity, positive predictive value and negative predictive value are calculated by means of the equations:

Table 8.1. Terminology of test results

Test	Disease status	Designation
+	+	True positive (a)
+	−	False positive (b)
−	+	False negative (c)
−	−	True negative (d)

$$
\begin{aligned}
\text{sensitivity} &= a/(a+c) \\
\text{specificity} &= d/(b+d) \\
\text{positive predictive value} &= a/(a+b) \\
\text{negative predictive value} &= d/(c+d)
\end{aligned}
$$

Moreover, the prevalence of the condition must be taken into consideration as must the question of whether arriving at a particular diagnosis will alter the clinical management such that other desired gains may offset patients' inconvenience, particularly those with negative results. This fine balance of factors attests to the quality of clinical practice. Clinicians, in fulfilling their obligations to their patients, will attempt to use the best available test to deduce the correct diagnosis, but are faced with the limitations imposed by the environment of managed care and rationalization of resources. This poses a moral dilemma to the clinician, where s/he has to calculate the worthiness of a life saved or a serious disease being missed.

ULTRASOUND SCAN

Technological advances over the last 30 years have established the use of ultrasound scanning in clinical gynecology, in particular the diagnosis of ovarian cysts and adnexal masses, and the management of ovulation-induction programs. Attempts at evaluation of the uterus have been successful where the uterine silhouette, uterine cervix and the endometrial thickness corresponding to the apposed endometrial surfaces are visualized[1,2]. Indeed, pelvic ultrasound scanning has become an integral part of modern gynecologic practice (Figure 8.1a).

Transvaginal ultrasound scanning of the pelvis adds a number of practical advantages, in particular obviating the need for a full bladder, which is mandatory in transabdominal scanning. Assessment of pelvic organs is made easier in cases of moderate obesity by using a vaginal probe, although in cases of severe obesity it may prove difficult to visualize the pelvic organs even with the transvaginal probe.

To assess the pelvic organs, the examiner should view the midline echo in the sagittal plane and move the ultrasound probe to image successive slices of the uterus on both sides of the midline. The maximum thickness of the midline echo of the double layer of the endometrium in the sagittal plane is measured, and any fluid within the uterine cavity is noted. Thereafter the uterus is examined in the coronal plane and successive images from the uterine cervix upward to the fundus

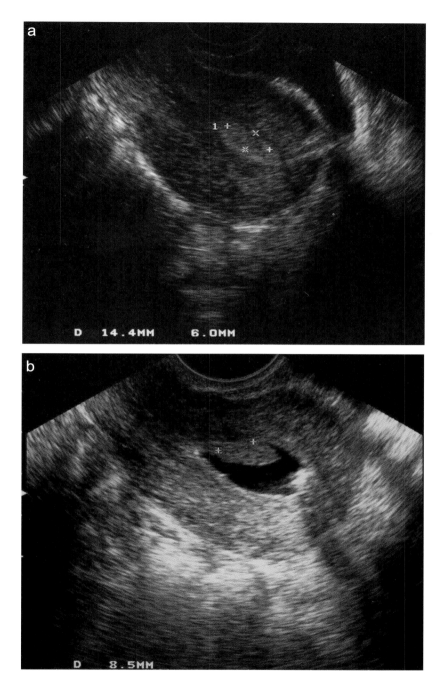

Figure 8.1. (**a**) Transvaginal ultrasound scan of the uterus showing endometrial echo; (**b**) saline instillation sonohysterography (SIS) showing an endometrial polyp. Courtesy of Mr N. Amso, University Hospital of Wales, Cardiff

127

are assessed. Only then can a three-dimensional picture of the uterine cavity be built up in the mind of the operator. In the case of a retroverted uterus, where the fundal region of the endometrium becomes less easy to evaluate, a head down tilt or a full bladder may help to raise the uterine fundus to within the detection range of the probe. Rapid technological developments in ultrasound scanning have seen the introduction of the three-dimensional composite images that help to facilitate the interpretation of the uterus and appendages as a whole. This technique awaits further clinical evaluation.

Color Doppler imaging has been tried in association with vaginal ultrasound scan to evaluate endometrial neovascularization, which presumably indicates a high risk of malignancy. In prospective studies of postmenopausal women, these findings did not add further information to that obtained by ultrasound scan alone and the technique did not discriminate between benign and malignant disease[3,4]. The ultrasound scan, therefore, helps to measure the size of the uterus and the endometrial thickness, and to identify the contrasting echoes of uterine fibroids or any fluid collection within the endometrial cavity. The examination must include an assessment of the ovaries to measure their size and the identification of any associated cystic lesion.

SALINE INSTILLATION SONOHYSTEROGRAPHY (SIS)

The instillation of a contrast medium into the uterine cavity using normal saline helps to delineate the presence of endometrial polyps and sometimes submucous fibroids as they distort the endometrial surface. After an initial ultrasound scan with the vaginal probe a bivalve speculum is introduced, the cervix is negotiated with a soft catheter, the speculum is removed, and finally the vaginal probe is reintroduced before 10 ml of sterile normal saline solution are injected into the uterus. Instillation of normal saline into the endometrial cavity helps to separate its anterior and posterior walls[5–8]. This technique is being increasingly used, particularly in premenopausal women, to detect intrauterine polyps, submucous fibroids and endometrial neoplasia. The procedure is associated with period-like pains due to the stimulation of uterine contractions. (Figure 8.1b). Further development of this technique has been reported recently using three-dimensional scanning of the uterine cavity following saline infusion. The images obtained were superior to those of the two-dimensional scans with saline infusion and have provided a more accurate diagnosis of focal endometrial polyps[9,10].

HYSTEROSCOPY

Panteleoni (1869) is credited as the first to describe the hysteroscope, but the clinical importance of hysteroscopy has been realized only during the last 2 decades, when developments in optics have made it possible to visualize the endometrium adequately and record the findings photographically, or by videotape, for further evaluation and comparison. Earlier reports described the use of the hysteroscope under general anesthesia; however, it is widely accepted that outpatient hysteroscopy with or without local anesthesia is a very well-tolerated procedure[11,12] and in experienced hands is just as accurate. Moreover it is easier to repeat when required, for example in cases of a recurrence of postmenopausal bleeding.

Panoramic hysteroscopy with CO_2 gas or fluid distension offers a direct visual examination of the whole of the endometrial cavity. It helps to identify the nature of endometrial abnormalities in terms of polyps, submucous fibroids and regional differences in endometrial thickness and its background color, as well as of the endometrial vascular pattern. Naked eye visualization through the hysteroscope offers a three-dimensional assessment of the uterine cavity and helps to assess the relationship between an identified abnormality and the general topography of the uterine cavity. The outer diameter of the instruments in common use ranges from 3.5 to 6 mm and, therefore, the need for cervical dilatation is limited. The disadvantage of using a gas distension medium is the formation of bubbles, especially in the presence of bleeding, which limits the view. By waiting for 30–60 seconds without manipulating the hysteroscope, these bubbles will burst. In addition, the escape of gas through the fallopian tubes may cause diaphragmatic irritation with pain typically referred to the tip of the shoulder. When this occurs, it is best to put the patient in a supine position for 5–10 minutes until the CO_2 gas is dissolved and absorbed by the peritoneal surfaces. Alternatively, and especially in the event of bleeding, distension of the uterus with normal saline can be used with pressure applied to the bag at 150 mmHg. This necessitates the use of a dual channel for irrigation and therefore cervical dilatation up to 8–9 mm may be required. The use of dextran 70 has been advocated and, since it is not miscible with blood, it may provide an excellent view. However, the possibility of allergic reactions and the potential for developing pulmonary edema if more than 300 ml are used have dampened initial enthusiasm for its application.

The use of closed circuit television systems is beneficial in allaying the patient's anxiety in an outpatient set-up, and is of immense educational value for trainees. However, its deployment may change the three-dimensional image to a two-dimensional one. The use of a beam splitter may help the examiner to overcome this where direct vision is maintained, with the camera still transmitting the endometrial images, but the beam splitter is notorious for reducing the amount of light available to the camera. New developments in three-dimensional camera systems may eliminate this difficulty.

Reported complications of outpatient hysteroscopy include vasovagal syncope, the incidence of which may be reduced by the subcutaneous injection of atropine 0.6 mg, given 10–15 minutes prior to the procedure. However, the incidence of vasovagal syncope in our unit, where we do not use atropine, has been 3 in 1000 and, therefore, it is difficult to justify its universal use. Reported postoperative infection is rare especially with CO_2 gas distension. Pregnancy is cited as a contraindication, but when abnormal bleeding is suspected to result from early pregnancy complications, measurement of β-human chorionic gonadotropin (β-HCG) level should preclude the use of the hysteroscope. The theoretical risk of disseminating uterine carcinoma has not been substantiated by any publication, and the biology of solid tumors is much more sophisticated than the simple seeding of exfoliating cells as a result of outpatient hysteroscopy. Air embolism may occur as a result of using a high gas flow rate under high pressure, and can be avoided by using hysteroflators equipped with pressure controls at 100 mmHg. All modern hysteroflators are designed to limit the gas flow rate to 100 ml/min, and the intrauterine pressure to a maximum of 200 mmHg. Perforation of the uterus does not occur when hysteroscopy is performed under local anesthesia, for the patient herself will safeguard against such rough handling (Figures 8.2 and 8.3).

ENDOMETRIAL BIOPSY

Ricci, in his excellent monograph on the history of gynecologic surgery and instruments, referred to Recamier in 1843 as the first to report the use of a small scoop attached to a long handle to remove fungal growths from the uterine cavity. He called the procedure 'curettage' and reported three deaths due to perforation and peritonitis[13]. The following 70 years witnessed conflicting attitudes toward this procedure. The optimization of the technique, the development of histologic criteria for diagnosis and the introduction of antisepsis made the deployment of uterine curettage an acceptable clinical practice in the early 20th century. Indeed, in 1925 Kelly recommended the carrying out of curettage as an office procedure without anesthesia[14].

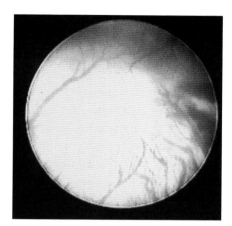

Figure 8.2. Hysteroscopic view of increased vascularity of the endometrium

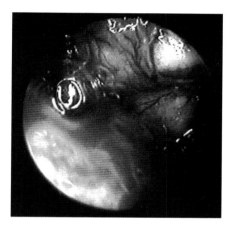

Figure 8.3. Hysteroscopic view of endometrial carcinoma showing grayish surface of the tumor and prominent vasculature

Reviews of large series of cases involving between 7000 and 21 000 women managed by dilatation of the cervix and curettage of the uterus (D&C) under general anesthesia appeared in the literature in which indications, accuracy and complications of the procedure were addressed[15,16]. In these series it was established that the risk of perforation of the uterus was about 1% . Endometrial diseases such as polyps, submucous fibroids, hyperplasia and carcinoma were missed in 7–10%, while endometrial cancer was detected in 17% of asymptomatic postmenopausal women. Nevertheless, these publications set the standard for all future developments in biopsy techniques, where D&C was repeatedly taken as the 'gold standard'.

The introduction of vacuum aspiration of endometrial tissue without anesthesia in 1970 heralded a new approach to endometrial sampling; this was subsequently called the Vabra aspirator[17]. It consists of a stainless steel cannula with a slightly curved tip, which has a wide slit at the concave aspect. The outer diameter of the cannula is 3 mm and it is attached to a plastic chamber encased by an outer plastic container. The latter is attached to a vacuum-generating electrical pump. A number of advantages have been cited for this technique, including high patient acceptability, feasibility of use by the clinician and a high concordance of histologic diagnosis of cancer when performed prior to hysterectomy. In a critical review of 33 published reports involving 13 598 D&C and 5851 Vabra aspirations, Grimes evaluated the accuracy and complication rates of these diagnostic procedures[18]. D&C is associated with mortality, and a high rate of postoperative hemorrhage and perforation compared to the Vabra curettage; no deaths have been reported with the use of the Vabra aspirator. When D&C or hysterectomy results were used to test the diagnostic accuracy of the Vabra aspirator, endometrial cancer was missed by the Vabra in 4% and endometrial polyps in 20% of instances[18].

Several tools have been invented to procure a sample of the endometrium, and the use of any of these instruments in an office setting may cause period-like cramps and discomfort. These tools embody the same principle as the Vabra, for instance using a plastic cannula instead of a metal one or using a syringe to replace the suction machine. A well-established device is the Pipelle de Cornier® endometrial sampler (Laboratoire CCD, Paris, France) which consists of a plastic cannula (about 3 mm outer diameter) with a slit at its tip. Suction is generated by an internal piston, which is pulled while rotating the cannula within the uterine cavity.

Having assessed the uterine cavity either by ultrasound scan or by office-based hysteroscopy, an endometrial biopsy is essential to establish a definitive histologic diagnosis. The cornerstone of the management of abnormal uterine bleeding in the peri- and postmenopause is the histologic assessment of the benignity of the endometrium and the exclusion of malignancy. The histopathologist can confidently report on the endometrial tissue recovered, which may or may not be representative of the rest of the endometrium. The limitations of routine endometrial sampling techniques in procuring tissue adequate for histologic examination are due to wide inter-operator variability, the technical difficulty in accessing the uterine cavity in up to 10% of postmenopausal women[19], and the fact that sampling of the endometrium causes pain. Therefore many clinical investigators attempt to equate the findings at ultrasound scan or SIS with the histologic features and set limits for endometrial thickness below which endometrial neoplasia is not likely to be present, thus justifying the omission of an endometrial biopsy. Cost-driven health care will no doubt compromise the accuracy of diagnosis, at least in some women.

The potential value of endometrial cytology in providing an alternative to endometrial biopsy and subsequent histologic assessment is severely limited and has not attracted much interest[20,21].

Effectiveness of the biopsy technique

Many authors have studied the sampling efficiency of various uterine samplers, and various comparisons have been reported in the literature. Pradhan and colleagues attempted to study the endometrium of premenopausal women presenting with cervical polyps by D&C under general anesthesia and reported failure to procure adequate samples for histologic assessment in 42% of cases. In a large multi-center study of women who were experiencing withdrawal bleeding while receiving sequential hormone replacement therapy (HRT), the endometrium was 'histologically not evaluable' in 27.1% of cases using the Pipelle de Cornier sampler[23], while the Vabra curet failed to procure a specimen in 18% of cases in another study[5]. Failure to reach the uterine cavity seems to be the main reason for the lack of an adequate endometrial sample. Another explanation was cited in a study by Rodriguez and colleagues[24], who found that the Pipelle device sampled about 4.2% of the total endometrial surface, compared to the sampling of 41.6% of the endometrium using the Vabra aspirator. Therefore a blind endometrial biopsy cannot reliably obtain a representative sample even when combined with ultrasound scan. A failed cancer detection rate of 4%[18] using the Vabra curet, and a discrepancy in diagnosis of up to 20% by hysterectomy, have dampened the initial enthusiasm for this technique[25,26].

The problem of assessing the endometrium in postmenopausal women was well illustrated by McBride, who reported a satisfactory specimen procurement rate of only 13% in 1521 women who had undergone D&C under general anesthesia[27], while a review of 141 consecutive cases of biopsies reported as 'insufficient for histological diagnosis' obtained from women with postmenopausal bleeding revealed 29 (20%) instances of uterine pathology after secondary investigation[28]. This underscores the importance of this clinical condition and the vigilance required in its investigation.

The success of aspiration methods in obtaining endometrial tissue adequate for diagnosis has been studied mainly in neoplastic states, where the friability of this tissue contributes greatly to the success of the sampling process. This is of significance for the majority of women who do not have a neoplastic endometrium, where the objective is to procure material for the diagnosis of functional endometrial changes, or when localized neoplasia involves a focus out of reach of the sampling device.

Site of the biopsy

In cases of menstrual disorders limited tissue procurement restricts the histologic interpretation of the findings and appropriate understanding of this dysfunctional

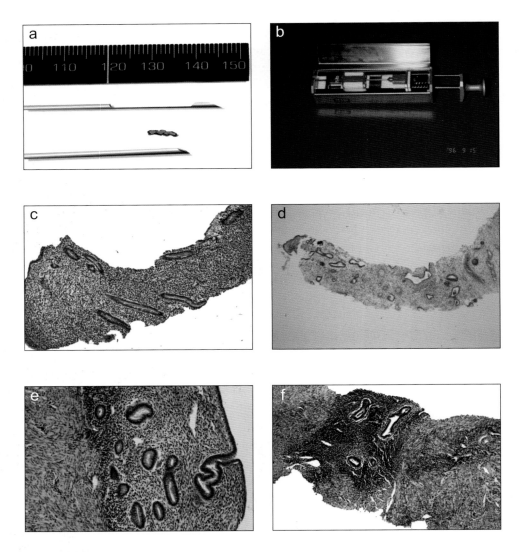

Figure 8.4. The Leicester Endometrial Needle Sampler (LENS). The tip of the needle biopsy and a typical sample (**a**) consists of a fine biopsy needle, housed within a cutting cannula (BIP; Biomed-Instrumente Produkte, Tårkenfeld, Germany). The LENS has a total length of 48 cm, and a diameter of 16G (1.6 mm). The sharp tipped needle or trocar is driven by a high-speed core cut device (**b**) to minimize tissue displacement and trauma. This is followed almost instantly by a similar thrust by the outer cutting cannula. Hematoxylin and eosin (H&E)-stained sections from the uterine fundus from cases with inactive postmenopausal endometrium (**c**), weakly proliferative endometrium (**d**), atrophic endometrium (**e**) and a case of adenomyosis (**f**). Reproduced with permission from the American College of Obstetricians and Gynecologists (Al-Azzawi F, Habiba M, Bell SC. *Obstet Gynecol* 1997;90:470–2[31])

problem. Regardless of the sampling instrument used, the tissue procured cannot be ascribed to a particular site of the endometrium, since it is a blind procedure, and regional variations of endometrial development have been widely documented[29,30]. Given the nature of the devices available, office procedures can only provide tissue from the superficial functionalis layer, and in the case of D&C under general anesthesia there is the risk of uterine perforation if deeper biopsies are sought. In addition, superficial biopsies cannot be oriented to enable the examination of the whole thickness vertically. Detailed information on the responsiveness of stromal tissue and the basalis layer of the endometrium, as well as the role of the cellular infiltration, during normal and abnormal menstruation is scant.

Other sampling devices

Hysteroscopically directed biopsy using biopsy forceps may procure site-specific samples, but such specimens are of limited depth, and in view of their size may become further degraded by fixation. The Leicester Endometrial Needle Sampler (LENS) has the advantage of obtaining a core biopsy specimen 1 mm in diameter and 12–16 mm deep, and as such it allows the examination of the whole thickness of the endometrium, including the endometrial–myometrial junctional zone (Figure 8.4)[31].

ACCEPTABILITY AND TOLERANCE

In evaluating the acceptability and tolerance of diagnostic techniques of the endometrium, the adjective 'invasive' is used to describe certain techniques. It carries a significant negative connotation which many authors have ascribed to hysteroscopy. Invasion is defined as infringement by intrusion, and to invade in the case of transvaginal ultrasound is the intrusion of the vaginal probe, while intrusion of the uterine cavity in the case of SIS and hysteroscopy is accomplished by the catheter and hysteroscope, respectively. Conceptually, there would be little difference between the two procedures had pain not been a factor to consider, but conventionally it is always applied to hysteroscopy. In many units intracervical infiltration of local anesthesia is used to facilitate the grasp and dilatation of the cervix[11,32] while other centers are able to provide a similar clinical service without local anesthesia[12,33]. Pain and discomfort during hysteroscopy or SIS may be due to uterine contractions in response to the distension medium but are more likely to be the result of endometrial biopsy.

In a prospective study using a visual analog scale, Downes and Al-Azzawi assessed pain and acceptability of outpatient hysteroscopy (using a 6-mm outer sheath) and endometrial biopsy using the vabra suction curet in postmenopausal women[11]. Of the first 100 women, only three expressed their preference for general anesthesia should subsequent examination with a hysteroscope be required. Seventy per cent of the women recorded a pain score below 5 (0 = no pain at all and 10 = the worst possible pain). When CO_2 gas distension is used a few women may experience shoulder tip pain, especially if the procedure is prolonged.

CHOICE OF METHOD OF INVESTIGATION

The choice of the method(s) of investigating the endometrium should be based on the objectives of that clinical encounter. If the question is purely whether the patient has endometrial neoplasia, then an adequate endometrial biopsy should suffice. If clinical evaluation of postmenopausal bleeding is required then the clinician is obliged to provide a thorough clinical assessment and full investigation of the reproductive system. Women who present to the gynecologist with abnormal bleeding expect a diagnosis of the highest standard rather than guesswork based on assessing the odds derived from the incidence of endometrial neoplasia in the general population. Cost containment is an important arbiter in deciding health policies, and as such it has encouraged a minimalist approach to investigation. This is further enhanced by the relatively low incidence of endometrial cancer (despite its being the fourth most common cancer in women), and the assumption that no serious 'harm' may be caused since the woman may bleed again anyway, if she happens to harbor a cancer.

The number of menopausal women is increasing, with the 'baby boomers' of the post-war years entering their sixth decade of life, and the problem of functional bleeding disorders may be encountered more often with the increase in HRT use. These functional bleeding disorders mandate effective methods of identifying endometrial polyps and submucous fibroids, since their removal is highly successful in rectifying abnormal bleeding while using HRT[34,35]. Moreover, appropriate and detailed evaluation of the endometrial histology may provide a guide to a corresponding adjustment in the dose of estrogen or progestogen.

In a comparative study, Fedele and colleagues[36] assessed the sensitivity and specificity of ultrasonography and hysteroscopy used in women with menstrual disorders and concluded that they were largely similar but that hysteroscopy was unsatisfactory in large cavities (six cases). Other workers have found that ultrasound scanning was inadequate to distinguish between polyps and fibroids[36–39]. Corson asserts that while ultrasound scan can be an accurate diagnostic tool for fibroids, only direct hysteroscopy can delineate the exact tumor location, shape, size and vascularity[40]. These are essential features that influence the decision as to whether a pharmacologic preparation of the uterus with gonadotropin-releasing hormone (GnRH) analog, for example, will be required prior to hysteroscopic myomectomy, and for the prediction of future bleeding patterns of postmenopausal women receiving sex steroid therapy[40].

The enthusiasm for ultrasound evaluation of the endometrium has prompted many investigators to test how safe it would be to forgo endometrial biopsy. The cut-off points in endometrial thickness have been tested and a 5-mm limit has been widely adopted[38,41]. A prerequisite of a clear symmetric endometrial echo of less than 5 mm encouraged Briley and Lindsell to omit endometrial biopsy[41]. Many reports, however, have shown that cancer cannot be excluded when endometrial thickness is below 5 mm, and have suggested 4- and 3-mm cut-off points instead[42–46]. Schramm and colleagues showed that the median endometrial thickness among uterine cancer patients was 4 mm, as opposed to 5.5 mm for those with atrophic endometrium, in a prospective evaluation of transvaginal ultrasound (TVU) compared to D&C as an independent procedure in 195 women presenting with spontaneous postmenopausal bleeding[47]. Endometrial cancer was detected in 29 women (15%). By adopting a cut-off point of ≥ 4 mm for endometrial thickness the sensitivity and specificity of TVU were 62% and 50%, respectively. Similar concerns were also reported in a series of 54 women who presented with spontaneous postmenopausal bleeding, where median endometrial thickness as measured by TVU was 5, 8.6 and 6 mm for histologically documented endometrial atrophy, hyperplasia and adenocarcinoma, respectively. Moreover, of the nine malignant samples, three cases had an endometrial thickness of 3 mm[48].

The SIS technique is claimed to provide accurate diagnosis of atrophic endometrium and endometrial polyps with sensitivities of 87.8 and 89.6% and specificities of 90.7 and 95%, respectively[49]. However, in this study SIS diagnosed only 40% of endometrial cancers, confirming the fundamental requirement for histologic examination of the endometrium in all cases. Soares and colleagues equated the accuracy of SIS to that of the 'gold standard' hysteroscopy and endometrial biopsy in the diagnosis of benign lesions – polyps, submucous fibroids and endometrial hyperplasia in premenopausal infertile women – but it failed to diagnose accurately intrauterine adhesions[50]. As a compromise, O'Connell and co-workers concluded that an office-based SIS with endometrial biopsy would be reliable enough in the management of postmenopausal bleeding when no endometrial abnormality was detected[51]. Where intrauterine luminal masses are suspected the patient should be referred for hysteroscopy and fractional curettage.

In one study of a series of 1398 women, 43% of whom were postmenopausal, diagnostic hysteroscopy and subsequent curettage confirmed that in addition to its being a basic tool in gynecologic practice, the sensitivity, specificity and global diagnostic precision of hysteroscopic evaluation of the endometrium are 100, 99.4 and 99.5%, respectively[52]. A similar experience was recorded with 980 women presenting with menstrual disorders[53], and with another series of 106 women who presented with postmenopausal bleeding[38], confirming the accuracy, safety and simplicity of outpatient hysteroscopy and endometrial sampling.

TRAINING

It may sound unnecessary to state that all diagnostic procedures require appropriate and adequate training programs. The fact remains that a high resolution and sophisticated ultrasound scanning machine is not a substitute for a skilled operator who can interpret the findings, an ability which is not acquired overnight. The procedure cannot be justified if the operator is not adequately cognizant of how to detect the presence of an adnexal mass, since to miss such pathology may have serious consequences for a patient's welfare. Similarly, office-based diagnostic hysteroscopy is operator-dependent, and appropriate training is fundamental. This issue is well illustrated by Schwarzler and colleagues, who evaluated the accuracy of transvaginal sonography (TVS), SIS and diagnostic hysteroscopy in 98 women aged 26–79 who failed to respond to initial medical treatment for abnormal uterine bleeding[54]. All these women subsequently underwent preoperative hysteroscopic assessment. Uterine abnormalities were detected in 53% of cases. The TVS and SIS techniques had sensitivities of 67 and 87%, specificities of 89 and 91%, positive predictive values of 88 and 92%, and negative predictive values of 71 and 86%, respectively. The sensitivity of diagnostic hysteroscopy was 90%; two cases with a polyp, two with a submucous fibroid and one with endometrial hyperplasia were not detected. The skill of the operator is demonstrated not only in identifying pathology, but also – and equally importantly – in negotiating the cervix and examining the whole uterine cavity without inflicting pain. The level of training extends to obtaining an endometrial biopsy, as one audit series, of 100 cases, indicated that registrars and residents are more likely to obtain an inadequate biopsy, and miss one of two cancer cases[55].

Given the nature and implications of postmenopausal bleeding, the concerns of the women affected are understandable. In the traditional setting, where clinical evaluation is performed in one department, ultrasound scan in another and further diagnostic procedures elsewhere, the delays involved and the necessity of meeting different personnel heighten the anxieties experienced by these women. The need for a comprehensive and precise work-up cannot be denied, but reducing the woman's anxiety can be accomplished by providing the whole service in a single setting where all procedures are conducted by the same gynecologist.

CLINICAL MANAGEMENT OF POSTMENOPAUSAL BLEEDING: ONE-STOP POSTMENOPAUSAL BLEEDING CLINIC

A detailed clinical history, including systems review and drug history, is essential to exclude conditions which may be the underlying cause of bleeding or which may influence subsequent management. A general physical examination (including the breasts) is required to establish normality, in particular a thorough abdominal examination to detect areas of tenderness, possible masses or ascites. Pelvic examination must be systematically conducted to exclude local vulvar, vaginal or cervical lesions. A smear for cytologic assessment is obtained, since the detection of abnormal squamous or glandular cells will be a clear indication for colposcopic assessment of the cervix and endometrial evaluation. A bimanual examination is performed to assess the overall uterine size, the mobility of the uterus and the characteristics of the supportive tissue. Bimanual examination also helps to exclude parametrial thickening, or adnexal masses.

Transvaginal ultrasound is performed to determine the size of the uterus, endometrial thickness and whether fluid exists within the endometrial cavity. The appendages are examined and any cystic lesion within the ovaries is measured. The size of the ovaries is measured and if they cannot be identified, this fact is noted. Any fluid in the pouch of Douglas is assessed and noted.

Panoramic hysteroscopy is performed, facilitated by four-quadrant intracervical injection of 4–6 ml of prilocaine 4%. The uterine cavity is measured by uterine sound, which helps to identify any difficulty in negotiating the cervical canal as a result of stenosis or cervical fibroids. Finally, a sample for endometrial biopsy is obtained using a Pipelle de Cornier sampler or the Vabra aspirator. A small sharp curet is occasionally used in some cases of tamoxifen-treated women. Should there be a localized lesion deemed not to have been adequately sampled, then the LENS device is used[31]. More than 1000 women have attended this clinic and further hysteroscopy under general anesthetic was needed in seven cases over 4 years. Our 'inadequate for histologic diagnosis' biopsy rate is less than 8% and in all these cases the endometrium was photographically documented as atrophic.

TREATMENT OF POSTMENOPAUSAL BLEEDING

If endometrial cancer is detected subsequent management is based on hysterectomy and bilateral removal of the uterine appendage. Subsequent radiotherapy is dependent on the tissue type, depth of invasion and extent of the tumor within the endometrium. The management of endometrial hyperplasia is largely dependent on the presence of atypia, which in postmenopausal women is best treated by hysterectomy, though a course of progestogen therapy is always worthwhile. Since the risk of carcinoma in cases of simple and complex hyperplasia without atypia is low, progestogen therapy for 3 months followed by repeat hysteroscopic evaluation and biopsy should be adequate for the majority of women, regardless of age, unless the woman insists on having a hysterectomy after thorough explanation and counseling.

The cytologic abnormality of 'atypical glandular cells of undetermined significance' (AGUS) is reported in 8–24 per 10 000 cervical smears. Cervical and/or uterine pathology has been detected in 20–72% of these women, depending on the intensity of the investigation[56,57]. This further emphasizes the importance of a full investigation of any episode of postmenopausal bleeding. Subsequent recurrence of postmenopausal bleeding demands equivalent vigilance in investigating the pelvic organs, despite a negative endometrial biopsy, cervical cytology or pelvic ultrasound scan obtained during the previous episode[58].

Where malignant disease is excluded, HRT in the form of combined sequential HRT is the treatment of choice. This may improve endometrial thickness and thus result in regular withdrawal bleeding. In cases of atrophic vaginitis and when systemic estrogen replacement treatment is contraindicated, estriol-based vaginal cream should provide adequate nourishment to the vaginal wall and improve the thickness of the lining squamous epithelium and the supporting collagen.

CONCLUSION

In patients presenting with menstrual disorders, unscheduled bleeding while under sex steroid treatment, spontaneous postmenopausal bleeding or bleeding as a result of tamoxifen therapy, adequate evaluation of the uterus is essential. It could be said that ultrasound scanning is an electronic extension of the gynecologic bimanual examination, aiding the evaluation of the size and structure of the pelvic organs. However, in examining the endometrium it does no more than provide a cut-off point, beyond which histologic abnormality is assumed to be infrequent or rare.

Following pelvic ultrasound scan, hysteroscopy is then performed and the process is concluded by the procurement of an adequate endometrial biopsy. Hysteroscopy is the only reliable tool to evaluate precisely the topography of the uterine cavity and the nature of the endometrium. It is the only realistic, and well tolerated, approach to targeting a suspected area of the endometrium, given the limitations of the currently available sampling devices; nonetheless it should be used along with ultrasound and endometrial biopsy in order to achieve a reliable diagnosis. Incomplete assessment leads to inappropriate treatment, which eventually frustrates patients and prompts many of them to opt for what is probably an unnecessary hysterectomy.

REFERENCES

1. Nakano H, Sakamoto C, Koyanagi T, Kubota S. Endometrial images by ultrasound. Nippon Sanka Fujinka Gakkai Zasshi. *Acta Obstet Gynaecol Japon* 1982;34:275–8
2. Fleischer AC, Kalemeris GC, Machin JE, *et al.* Sonographic depiction of normal and abnormal endometrium with histopathologic correlation. *J Ultrasound Med* 1986;5:445–52
3. Chan FY, Chau MT, Pun TC, *et al.* Limitations of transvaginal sonography and color Doppler imaging in the differentation of endometrial carcinoma from benign lesions. *J Ultrasound Med* 1994;13:623–8
4. Vuento MH, Pirhonen JP, Makinen JI, *et al.* Screening for endometrial cancer in asymptomatic postmenopausal women with conventional and colour Doppler sonography. *Br J Obstet Gynaecol* 1999;106:14–20
5. Goldstein SR, Nachtigall M, Snyder JR, Nachtigall L. Endometrial assessment by vaginal ultrasonography before endometrial sampling in patients with postmenopausal bleeding. *Am J Obstet Gynecol* 1990;163:119–23

6. Parsons AK, Lense JJ. Sonohysterography for endometrial abnormalities: preliminary results. *J Clin Ultrasound* 1993;21:87–95

7. Dubinsky TJ, Parvey HR, Gormaz G, *et al.* Transvaginal hysterosonography: comparison with biopsy in the evaluation of postmenopausal bleeding. *J Ultrasound Med* 1995;14:887–93

8. Cicinelli E, Romano F, Anastasio PS, *et al.* Sonohysterography versus hysteroscopy in the diagnosis of endouterine polyps. *Gynecol Obstet Invest* 1994;38:266–71

9. Bonilla-Musoles F, Raga F, Osborne NG, *et al.* Three-dimensional hysterosonography for the study of endometrial tumors: comparison with conventional transvaginal sonography, hysterosalpingography, and hysteroscopy. *Gynecol Oncol* 1997;65:245–52

10. La Torre R, De Felice C, De Angelis C, *et al.* Transvaginal sonographic evaluation of endometrial polyps: a comparison wth two dimensional and three dimensional contrast sonography. *Clin Exp Obstet Gynecol* 1999;26:171–3

11. Downes E, Al-Azzawi F. How well do perimenopausal patients accept outpatient hysteroscopy? Visual analogue scoring of acceptability and pain in 100 women. *Eur J Obstet Gynecol Reprod Biol* 1993;48:37–41

12. Broadbent JA, Hill NC, Molnar BG, *et al.* Randomized placebo controlled trial to assess the role of intracervical lignocaine in outpatient hysteroscopy. *Br J Obstet Gynaecol* 1992;99:777–9

13. Ricci JV. Gynaecological surgery and instruments of the nineteenth century prior to the antiseptic age. In Ricci JV. *The Development of Gynaecological Surgery and Instruments.* Philadelphia: Blackiston, 1949:326–8

14. Kelly HA. Curettage without anesthesia on the office table. *Am J Obstet Gynecol* 1925;9:78

15. Ward B, Gravlee LC, Wideman GL. The fallacy of simple uterine curettage. *Obstet Gynecol* 1958;12:642

16. Hofmeister FJ. Endometrial biopsy: another look. *Am J Obstet Gynecol* 1974;118:773

17. Jensen JG. Vacuum curettage. *Danish Med Bull* 1970;17:199

18. Grimes DA. Diagnostic dilation and curettage: a reappraisal. *Am J Obstet Gynecol* 1982;142:1–6

19. Van den Bosch T, Vandendael A, Van Schoubroeck D, *et al.* Combining vaginal ultrasonography and office endometrial sampling in the diagnosis of endometrial disease in postmenopausal women. *Obstet Gynecol* 1995;85:349–52

20. Koonings PP, Moyer DL, Grimes DA. A randomized clinical trial comparing Pipelle and Tis-u-trap for endometrial biopsy. *Obstet Gynecol* 1990;75:293–5

21. Van den Bosch T, Vandendael A, Wranz PA, Lombard CJ. Endopap- versus Pipelle-sampling in the diagnosis of postmenopausal endometrial disease. *Eur J Obstet Gynecol Reprod Biol* 1996;64:91–4

22. Pradhan S, Chenoy R, O'Brien PM. Dilatation and curettage in patients with cervical polyps: a retrospective analysis. *Br J Obstet Gynaecol* 1995;102:415–17

23. Sturdee DW, Barlow DH, Ulrich LG, *et al.* Is the timing of withdrawal bleeding a guide to endometrial safety during sequential oestrogen–progestagen replacement therapy? UK Continuous Combined HRT Study Investigators [published erratum appears in *Lancet* 1994;344(8935):1516]. *Lancet* 1994;344:979–82

24. Rodriguez GC, Yaqub N, King ME. A comparison of the Pipelle device and the Vabra aspirator as measured by endometrial denudation in hysterectomy specimens: the

Pipelle device samples significantly less of the endometrial surface than the Vabra aspirator. *Am J Obstet Gynecol* 1993;168:55–9

25. Denis R Jr, Barnett JM, Forbes SE. Diagnostic suction curettage. *Obstet Gynecol* 1973; 42:301–3

26. Webb MJ, Gaffey TA. Outpatient diagnostic aspiration curettage. *Obstet Gynecol* 1976; 47:239–42

27. McBride JM. The normal postmenopausal endometrium. *J Obstet Gynaecol Br Emp* 1954;61:691–7

28. Farrell T, Jones N, Owen P, Baird A. The significance of an 'insufficient' Pipelle sample in the investigation of post-menopausal bleeding. *Acta Obstet Gynecol Scand* 1999;78:810–12

29. Dallenbach-Hellweg G, Poulsen H, eds. *Atlas of Endometrial Histopathology.* New York: Springer, 1996:105–9

30. Shaw ST Jr, Macaulay LK, Hohman WR. Vessel density in endometrium of women with and without intrauterine contraceptive devices: a morphometric evaluation. *Am J Obstet Gynecol* 1979;135:202–6

31. Al-Azzawi F, Habiba M, Bell SC. The Leicester Endometrial Needle Sampler: a novel device for endometrial and myometrial junctional zone biopsy. *Obstet Gynecol* 1997;90: 470–2

32. Zupi E, Luciano AA, Valli E, *et al.* The use of topical anesthesia in diagnostic hysteroscopy and endometrial biopsy. *Fertil Steril* 1995;63:414–16

33. Vercellini P, Colombo A, Mauro F, *et al.* Paracervical anesthesia for outpatient hysteroscopy. *Fertil Steril* 1994;62:1083–5

34. Al-Azzawi F. Prediction of successful outcome following hysteroscopic laser myomectomy in women with heavy and unscheduled bleeding. *Climacteric* 1999;2(Suppl):289

35. Cravello L, de Montgolfier R, D'Ercole C, *et al.* Hysteroscopic surgery in postmenopausal women. *Acta Obstet Gynecol Scand* 1996;75:563–6

36. Fedele L, Bianchi S, Dorta M, *et al.* Transvaginal ultrasonography versus hysteroscopy in the diagnosis of uterine submucous myomas. *Obstet Gynecol* 1991;77:745–8

37. Hulka CA, Hall DA, McCarthy K, Simeone JF. Endometrial polyps, hyperplasia, and carcinoma in postmenopausal women: differentiation with endovaginal sonography. *Radiology* 1994;191:755–8

38. Loverro G, Bettocchi S, Cormio G, *et al.* Transvaginal sonography and hysteroscopy in postmenopausal uterine bleeding. *Maturitas* 1999;33:139–44

39. Cacciatore B, Ramsay T, Lehtovirta P, Ylostalo P. Transvaginal sonography and hysteroscopy in postmenopausal bleeding. *Acta Obstet Gynecol Scand* 1994;73:413–16

40. Corson SL. Hysteroscopic diagnosis and operative therapy of submucous myoma. *Obstet Gynecol Clin North Am* 1995;22:739–55

41. Briley M, Lindsell DR. The role of transvaginal ultrasound in the investigation of women with post-menopausal bleeding. *Clin Radiol* 1998;53:502–5

42. Bakour SH, Dwarakanath LS, Khan KS, *et al.* The diagnostic accuracy of ultrasound scan in predicting endometrial hyperplasia and cancer in postmenopausal bleeding. *Acta Obstet Gynecol Scand* 1999;78:447–51

43. Karlsson B, Granberg S, Wikland M, *et al.* Transvaginal ultrasonography of the endometrium in women with postmenopausal bleeding – a Nordic multicenter study. *Am J Obstet Gynecol* 1995;172:1488–94

44. Kekre AN, Jose R, Seshadri L. Transvaginal sonography of the endometrium in south Indian postmenopausal women. *Aust N Z J Obstet Gynaecol* 1997;37: 449–51

45. Granberg S, Ylostalo P, Wikland M, Karlsson B. Endometrial sonographic and histologic findings in women with and without hormonal replacement therapy suffering from postmenopausal bleeding. *Maturitas* 1997;27:35–40

46. Guner H, Tiras MB, Karabacak O, *et al.* Endometrial assessment by vaginal ultrasonography might reduce endometrial sampling in patients with postmenopausal bleeding: a prospective study. *Aust N Z J Obstet Gynaecol* 1996;36:175–8

47. Schramm T, Kurzl R, Schweighart C, Stuckert-Klein AC. [Endometrial carcinoma and vaginal ultrasound: studies of the diagnostic validity.] *J Geburtshilfe Frauenheilkd* 1995; 55:65–72

48. Buyuk E, Durmusoglu F, Erenus M, Karakoc B. Endometrial disease diagnosed by transvaginal ultrasound and dilatation and curettage. *Acta Obstet Gynecol Scand* 1999;78: 419–22

49. Bernard JP, Lecuru F, Darles C, *et al.* Saline contrast sonohysterography as first-line investigation for women with uterine bleeding. *Ultrasound Obstet Gynecol* 1997;10:121–5

50. Soares SR, Barbosa dos Reis MM, Camargos AF. Diagnostic accuracy of sonohysterography, transvaginal sonography, and hysterosalpingography in patients with uterine cavity diseases. *Fertil Steril* 2000;73:406–11

51. O'Connell LP, Fries MH, Zeringue E, Brehm W. Triage of abnormal postmenopausal bleeding: a comparison of endometrial biopsy and transvaginal sonohysterography versus fractional curettage with hysteroscopy. *Am J Obstet Gynecol* 1998;178:956–61

52. Torrejon R, Fernandez-Alba JJ, Carnicer I, *et al.* The value of hysteroscopic exploration for abnormal uterine bleeding. *J Am Assoc Gynecol Laparosc* 1997;4:453–6

53. Loverro G, Bettocchi S, Cormio G, *et al.* Diagnostic accuracy of hysteroscopy in endometrial hyperplasia. *Maturitas* 1996;25:187–91

54. Schwarzler P, Concin H, Bosch H, *et al.* An evaluation of sonohysterography and diagnostic hysteroscopy for the assessment of intrauterine pathology. *Ultrasound Obstet Gynecol* 1998;11:337–42

55. Gordon SJ, Westgate J. The incidence and management of failed Pipelle sampling in a general outpatient clinic. *Aust N Z J Obstet Gynaecol* 1999;39:115–18

56. Kim TJ, Kim HS, Park CT, *et al.* Clinical evaluation of follow-up methods and results of atypical glandular cells of undetermined significance (AGUS) detected on cervicovaginal Pap smears. *Gynecol Oncol* 1999;73:292–8

57. Cheng RF, Hernandez E, Anderson LL, *et al.* Clinical significance of a cytologic diagnosis of atypical glandular cells of undetermined significance. *J Reprod Med* 1999; 44:922–8

58. Feldman S, Shapter A, Welch WR, Berkowitz RS. Two-year follow-up of 263 patients with post/perimenopausal vaginal bleeding and negative initial biopsy. *Gynecol Oncol* 1994;55:56–9

9
Management of the menopause
F. Al-Azzawi

DIAGNOSIS OF THE MENOPAUSE

The majority of postmenopausal women who present to their doctors requesting help suffer from hot flushes, sweating and vaginal dryness, though a few present wishing to prevent osteoporosis or ischemic heart disease. The clinical diagnosis of the menopause depends on the presence of typical symptoms and/or amenorrhea for more than 12 months.

Shortening of the follicular phase is responsible for the majority of short menstrual cycles, where the luteal phase remains relatively constant. Clinically, this may present as a mixed picture of vasomotor symptoms, menstrual irregularity, breast tenderness and emotional lability that appears 7–10 days postmenstruum. Premature corpus luteum failure may present as premenstrual blood loss in the form of spotting or brown discharge for 3–4 days before frank menstruation occurs. This erratic ovarian responsiveness is more frequent during the 4 years preceding the menopause than during the years of menstrual maturity[1].

In women who are still menstruating, the differential diagnosis includes the premenstrual syndrome, especially when associated with symptoms of the climacteric. Endogenous depression is another consideration in the differential diagnosis. Sometimes vasomotor symptoms are part of rare or infrequent conditions such as pheochromocytoma or hyperthyroidism, but other features of these conditions and the characteristic biochemical changes may establish the relevant diagnosis.

Amenorrhea

The diagnosis of the menopause is easy when one knows that the last menstrual period is the final menstrual event, and therefore it is a retrospective diagnosis.

This was illustrated by Wallace and colleagues[2], where over 5000 women were grouped in age ranges 45–49, 50–52 and ≥ 53 years of age. The occurrence of menstrual bleeding after episodes of amenorrhea of up to 1 year was calculated (Figure 9.1). Even after 6 months of amenorrhea a further menstrual episode can be anticipated in 45–72% of instances, depending on the woman's age.

Hormonal assays

Abrupt cessation of ovarian function may occur in 20% of women where a low estradiol level, of < 50 pmol/l, and raised follicle-stimulating hormone (FSH), > 30 IU/l, can be documented. More commonly, however, the decline in ovarian function may show elevations of FSH level but estradiol may still be produced at normal levels. Measurements of FSH and estradiol levels are not required for routine diagnosis, but they may be of help in establishing the diagnosis of ovarian failure in atypical cases, in the follow-up of incomplete response to treatment, or in the case of conserved ovaries following hysterectomy. A low serum inhibin B level may help in the assessment of ovarian folliculogenesis[3], but the assay requires further evaluation before it can be recommended for clinical practice.

Assessment of ovarian reserve has been attempted to predict the diagnosis of the menopause using the clomiphene citrate challenge test[4], or gonadotropin-releasing hormone agonist test[5], but none of these functional tests has been shown to be reliable enough to adopt clinically[6].

TREATMENT OF THE MENOPAUSE

The principle of hormone replacement therapy (HRT) involves the administration of estrogen, which provides relief of symptoms, reverses the changes in calcium handling and bone remodeling, and improves lipoprotein metabolism. Estradiol and estrone are fat-soluble molecules and therefore not readily absorbed from the gut unless the steroid is micronized (particle size < 1 μm), or if the estrogens are esterified to a carrier ester that makes them more water-soluble. An example of the latter is estradiol valerate, which is quickly metabolized in the liver into estradiol and valeric acid, a 12-C fatty acid. Ethinylestradiol is another example, but because of its resistance to degradation by the intracellular 17β-dehydrogenase it exerts a sustained activity, and therefore has become less popular for postmenopausal HRT.

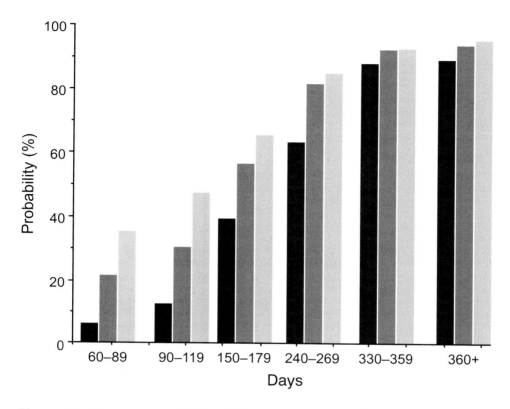

Figure 9.1. Percentage probability of the menopause according to the duration of amenorrhea. Data from Wallace RB, Sherman BM, Bean JA, *et al. Am J Obstet Gynecol* 1979;135:1021–4. ■ , 45–49 years; ▦ , 50–52 years; ▨ , ≥ 53 years

Oral administration of estrogen is subjected to the first pass effect of the liver, with rapid conversion of estradiol to the weaker estrone and subsequent conjugation to glucuronates and sulfates. The impact on the liver is demonstrated by increased hepatic globin synthesis. Oral therapy usually succeeds in building up satisfactory serum estradiol levels. The transdermal preparations offer a theoretically safer way to administer estrogen, where the hepatic first pass effect is reduced, but suffer from limitations of skin absorption in at least 50% of instances, and the potential for skin reactions to the adhesive material of the patch. The application of estradiol in gel formulation rubbed over the skin may overcome the problem of skin irritation; nevertheless, serum estradiol levels may still be lower than those achievable with oral therapy. The subcutaneous insertion of estradiol pellets involves a surgical procedure and is associated with high serum estradiol levels; as such it is responsible for the development of tachyphylaxis in a significant number of women. The vaginal route is effective in delivering estrogen when a restricted effect to the vagina is required, but the frequent application of vaginal creams and pessaries may sometimes deliver enough estrogen to stimulate the uterus and cause vaginal bleeding, an important consideration in the differential diagnosis of post-menopausal bleeding. The significance of the route of administration of estrogen and the consequences of the first pass effect on hepatic metabolism were challenged by Goebelsmann and colleagues[7], when hepatic globin synthesis was taken as a marker of the hepatic first pass effect. They found that the net effect on the synthesis of hepatic globin was a function of the serum level of the estrogens administered and not the route of administration.

New developments in parenteral routes of administration

The active development of novel and effective parenteral delivery systems which address the issues of frequency of administration and the need to maintain the principle of steady state kinetics has been successful. An estradiol-impregnated vaginal ring, which delivers adequate amounts of estradiol and requires changing every 10–12 weeks, is currently under development. A nasal spray has been developed for estradiol administration. It characteristically results in a surge of estradiol with return to the baseline after 3–4 hours. Its efficacy in relieving symptoms of estrogen deficiency is similar to those of orally or transdermally used systems. In combination with sequential progestogens it resulted in a bleeding pattern and endometrial histologic changes similar to those of estradiol–progestogen continuously administered through other routes. Whether this method of delivery offers a better long-term clinical efficacy remains to be seen[8].

Adverse effects of estrogens

Adverse effects of estrogens are:

(1) Nausea and gastric irritation (which may be caused by oral preparations);

(2) Breast tenderness, usually dose-related, which generally settles down within 3–4 months;

(3) Headaches; and

(4) Skin irritation (which can be caused by transdermal preparations).

Other adverse effects include weight changes, water retention, rashes and chloasma, changes in liver enzymes, depression and leg cramps.

The average daily doses of estrogen depicted in Table 9.1 are derived from the literature for the provision of adequate control of vasomotor symptoms. The dose of estrogen may be increased to overcome residual vasomotor symptoms. Nevertheless, a minimum level of 100 pmol/l of estradiol is required for effective protection against postmenopausal bone loss[9].

The need for a progestogen

The continuous administration of estrogen causes progressive proliferation of the endometrium. Such stimulation may lead to the development of endometrial hyperplasia, or even carcinoma of the endometrium[10], and therefore estrogen-only therapy can be given safely only to women who have had a hysterectomy. Over the last 40 years progestogens have been introduced to offset the effect of stimulation of the endometrium by continuous estrogen. A progestogen is administered cyclically, for 12–14 days every month, and this regimen is usually followed by menstrual discharge. Alternatively, the progestogen may be used continuously alongside the estrogen, the aim being to induce amenorrhea. There is a wide variation in bioavailability and individual tissue concentrations of different progestogens, making it difficult to derive relative potencies between various compounds. Moreover, the variation of the incidence and severity of adverse effects between different individuals necessitates an individual approach to treatment in terms of both dose and type of progestogen (Chapter 5).

The choice of progestogen may be influenced by cycle control. Levonorgestrel offers better cycle control, for example, compared to norethisterone, while the incidence of intermenstrual bleeding may be even less with gestodene-containing preparations[11].

Tibolone

Tibolone, a synthetic steroid – $(7\alpha,17\alpha)$-17-hydroxy-7-methyl-19-norpregn-5 (10)-en-20-yn-3-one (Livial®, Organon, UK) – is a 'gonadomimetic' steroid with combined weak progestogenic, weak estrogenic and weak androgenic properties. It may be used alone or as a supplement for postmenopausal women to treat

Table 9.1. Drugs used for postmenopausal hormone replacement therapy (HRT)

	Type	Average daily dose
Estrogen		
Oral	Micronized estradiol	2 mg
	Conjugated estrogens	0.625 mg
	Estradiol valerate	2 mg
	Piperazine estrone sulfate	0.625 mg
Transdermal	Estradiol in adhesive matrix or reservoir patch	50 µg
	Estradiol in a gel formulation	2.5 g
Subcutaneous pellets*		50 mg
Vaginal applications	Dienestrol cream	These are administered daily for 3 weeks followed by twice-weekly administration to minimize unopposed estrogen effect on the uterus
	Estriol cream	
	Estradiol vaginal tablets	
	Conjugated equine estrogens cream	
*Progestational agents***	Micronized progesterone	300 mg
	19-Nortestosterone derivatives	
	Norethisterone (norethindrone)	1 mg
	Levonorgestrel	0.075 mg
	Norgestrel	0.150 mg
	C-21 derivatives of progesterone	
	Medroxyprogesterone acetate	10 mg
	Dydrogesterone	10–20 mg
	Trimegestone	0.5 mg
Other synthetic compounds	Tibolone	2.5 mg
	Raloxifene	60 mg

*Subcutaneous pellets are administered at 6-monthly intervals; **the average daily dose of progestational agents refers to sequential regimens vasomotor symptoms and to reduce postmenopausal bone loss. The rate of increase in bone mineral density is estimated at about 3–4% per year, which is comparable to that of estrogens[12–15]. It may help to alleviate vasomotor symptoms without causing mastalgia, but is also associated in some women with the development of bloating, fluid retention and psychologic symptoms similar to those of premenstrual tension. It is administered orally in a daily dose of 2.5 mg. Tibolone provides an amenorrheic regimen and does not cause uterine bleeding in the majority of users. Nevertheless, the occurrence of bleeding should be investigated as in any case of spontaneous postmenopausal bleeding. Six cases of endometrial hyperplasia and adenocarcinoma in patients on tibolone treatment have been reported, all of whom presented with vaginal bleeding. It is significant that two out of the four women who had endometrial cancer in that series also had other significant risk factors for cancer: one was obese and the other had been on unopposed estrogen for 15 years. Neither of these women had confirmatory normal biopsies prior to commencing therapy. In that series the diagnosis of endometrial hyperplasia was made in two cases, both of whom were diagnosed as having endometrial hyperplasia in an endometrial polyp, while the rest of the endometrium was either atrophic or reported as normal[16]. In another series of women who presented with bleeding while being treated with tibolone, a higher incidence (27%) of endometrial polyps was noted[17]. However, immunohistochemical evaluation of the recovered endometrium using anti-Ki-67 antibodies did not show higher endometrial proliferative activity in those who bled on tibolone compared to those who did not[18].

The influence of tibolone on lipid metabolism has been investigated. Total cholesterol is reduced as a result of treatment, the high-density lipoprotein (HDL)-cholesterol level being reduced more profoundly compared to the continuous combined HRT regimen[19]. These observations confirm earlier reports, which documented the significant lowering effect of two doses of tibolone (1.25 mg and 2.5 mg daily) on HDL-cholesterol and a corresponding lowering of apolipoprotein AI. There was no lowering effect on low-density lipoprotein (LDL)-cholesterol, apolipoprotein B or lipoprotein(a). Serum total cholesterol and triglyceride levels were, nevertheless, reduced[20]. The two dose levels of tibolone resulted in a similar, marked lowering (30%) of tissue plasminogen activator and plasminogen activator inhibitor activity as compared with placebo, while plasminogen was increased (15%) in both groups. Whether the beneficial changes in markers of fibrinolysis and coagulation would effectively offset the adverse effects on HDL-cholesterol remain to be seen. These adverse lipid effects were further documented when tibolone and a combined regimen of oral estradiol valerate with intramuscularly administered dihydroandrosterone enanthate were compared with transdermal estradiol alone[21].

With these provisos in mind, tibolone is indicated in women who have passed the menopause, who do not wish to bleed or in those with contraindications to the use of estrogen.

Raloxifene

Selective estrogen receptor modulators (SERMs) are a family of compounds found to exert estrogenic effects in certain body tissues but not in others. Raloxifene, a non-steroidal benzothiaphene, is chemically related to tamoxifen. Both raloxifene and tamoxifen bind the estrogen receptors and show mixed agonist and antagonist activity in different estrogen-responsive tissues. Both drugs reduce bone turnover and modulate hepatic globin synthesis, in a manner similar to estrogen. Raloxifene, however, does not stimulate the uterus, unlike tamoxifen, which acts as a partial estrogen agonist on the uterus. Raloxifene is orally administered as a daily dose of 60 mg, and is metabolized by the liver and undergoes extensive enterohepatic cycling.

Raloxifene has been shown to reduce markers of bone turnover and may result in an increase of vertebral bone mineral density by about 1.2–1.6% per annum[22] and therefore it is less effective than estrogen. However, there are no bone data directly comparing the two treatments. There appears to be no endometrial stimulatory effect of raloxifene compared to controls, in terms of endometrial thickness measured by ultrasound or the incidence of uterine bleeding[23]. Raloxifene may reduce serum cholesterol and LDL-cholesterol levels, similarly to HRT, but it does not affect the HDL-cholesterol levels or the triglycerides, which rise by 11–20% with HRT[24].

Raloxifene seems to be devoid of breast stimulatory effects and claims have been made of a lower propensity to develop new breast cancers during treatment for up to 3 years[25]. However, there is an increase in the incidence of vasomotor symptoms with raloxifene treatment. There is an increased risk of thromboembolism, to the same extent as that of HRT, and also leg cramps. Clearly this preparation is indicated in women who have passed the menopause, who do not complain of vasomotor symptoms and who are at an increased risk of osteoporosis. It may prove useful in the prevention and treatment of osteoporosis, as an alternative to HRT, in women with estrogen-dependent neoplasia and those who do not wish to bleed.

HRT AND COMPLIANCE

No more than 50–60% of women will continue to take HRT beyond 1 year and one of the main causes of non-compliance with HRT in peri- and postmenopausal women is withdrawal bleeding, particularly if irregular or heavy. Progestogenic side-effects adversely affect compliance, but manipulation of the dose and type of progestogen may help to ameliorate this problem. However, attempts to minimize the progestogenic adverse effects by reducing the dose of the progestogen may jeopardize cycle control. This issue is further discussed in Chapter 2. Other factors that affect compliance include weight gain, fear of cancer and risk of thromboembolism.

Weight gain

Increase in body weight is a recognized feature during the fifth decade in many women and central fat deposition becomes more pronounced after the meno-pause[26–28]. Whether weight gain is due to declining physical activity with unchanged calorie intake, or to deterioration of ovarian activity remains unknown. It is plausible to attribute postmenopausal deposition of abdominal fat to the relative hyperandrogenic state resulting from continued stromal production of androgens together with estrogen deficiency, the hallmark of the menopause. Regardless of its etiology, weight gain is a function of calorie intake.

Increased body weight, particularly central abdominal fat deposition, is a recognized risk factor for cardiovascular disease and type II diabetes mellitus. Positive correlations have been identified between excess weight and endometrial cancer[29], breast cancer[30] and colorectal cancer[31]. The issue of excess weight and the incidence of cancer is related to a number of factors such as total calories, type of fat and type and amount of protein consumed. On the other hand, negative correlations with cancer risk were identified, including fruit and vegetable intake and a high level of physical activity[32].

Weight gain as a result of taking HRT is a common complaint among women; however, all available data suggest that the weight gain is no different from that in untreated groups[33]. Control of fluid retention and craving for sugar can sometimes be achieved by changing the type of progestogen or increasing the dose of estrogen, particularly in women with residual menopausal symptoms. Dieting alone is not adequate to lose weight, and physical exercise – at gradually increasing intensity – should be encouraged. Not only does exercise reduce cardiovascular risk and increase the HDL-cholesterol level, but it also lessens the impact of dieting on muscle mass.

The risk of breast cancer

In the Western world cancer of the breast is the leading type of cancer in women and is the second leading cause of cancer deaths[34]. Its incidence rises sharply between the ages of 50 and 60. It is a multifactorial condition and its etiologic relationship to estrogen therapy has long been suggested but never proven. Concern about its relationship with estrogen is the most commonly stated reason for discontinuation of HRT. An increased relative risk of breast cancer in women receiving estrogen replacement therapy (ERT) was postulated to be around 1.45 (95% confidence interval (CI), 1.22–1.74) for 5–9 years of use and 1.46 (95% CI, 1.20–1.76) for 10 or more years of use, but past users were not shown to be at an increased risk. Given the size of the Nurses' Health Study and the quality of analysis, these data are perhaps the strongest available[35]. However, detection bias cannot be discounted, since the mammography rate in hormone users was 14% higher than in non-users, with a reproductive history suggestive of high-risk attributes, such as early menarche at less than 13 years and low parity. Nonetheless, the association of higher breast cancer risk with HRT use was refuted by others[36–40]. Furthermore, there was no observed increase in the risk of breast cancer or its mortality in the Iowa Women's Health Study after 8 years of follow-up, even in those women with a family history of breast cancer[41]. The addition of progestogens, as a sequential or continuous combined regimen with estrogen to offset the endometrial effects of the latter, has not been shown to offer protection against breast cancer[42]. Nevertheless, when counseling women who wish to commence HRT, all these issues should be discussed and the data should be presented in a manner understandable by the patient (Figure 9.2)[43,44].

Women should be advised on breast self-examination on a monthly basis, and to have a breast examination annually by their doctor or practice nurse. Although this may result in increasing referrals to breast units with the attendant anxieties while awaiting the results of investigations, it is in the author's view a fundamental part of a 'breast awareness' campaign. Screening mammography is currently performed in the UK every 3 years between the ages of 50 and 64, but 25% of 'interval' cancers not identified at screening occur between the second and third year. Therefore, particularly in high-risk women, mammography is advised at least every 2 years. Data on mammography screening which were started at the age of 45 and performed at 2-year intervals resulted in a 25% reduction in mortality after 14 years of

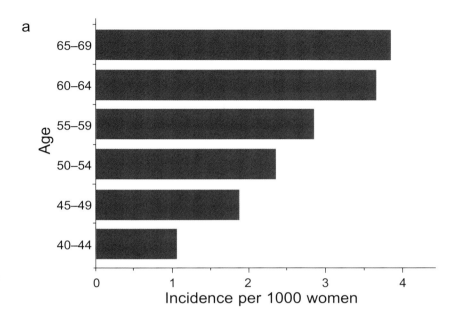

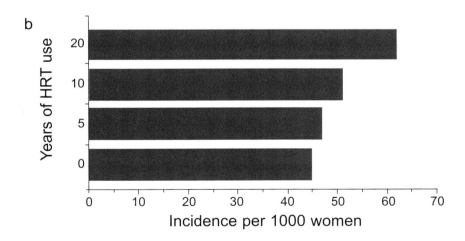

Figure 9.2. (a) Age-related incidence of breast cancer; overall incidence of 2255 cases in 947 468 women, non-screened population; (b) incidence of breast cancer per 1000 women (users and non-users of hormone replacement therapy (HRT)) between 50 and 70 years of age. (Non-users of HRT are denoted by '0 years'.) Data from (a) Danish National Board of Health (Copenhagen: Sunhedsstyrelsen, 1999)[43]; and (b) Collaborative Group on Hormonal Factors in Breast Cancer. *Lancet* 1997;350:1047–59[44]

follow-up[45]. These data are in agreement with most meta-analyses of randomized trials[46].

Risk of endometrial cancer

The use of unopposed estrogen, cyclically or continuously administered, promotes endometrial mitotic activity and results in hyperplasia, simple and complex, and early carcinoma of the endometrium. After 1 year of treatment the incidence of hyperplasia is increased by 20%[47]. The average time for progression of hyperplasia to carcinoma of the endometrium is about five years, and 25–30% of atypical hyperplasia progress to carcinoma within 1 year[48]. In a recent case–control study from Sweden the relative risk of developing endometrial carcinoma after 5 or more years of use of unopposed estrogen was markedly increased, for estradiol (odds ratio (OR) = 6.2; 95% CI, 3.6–12.0) and for conjugated equine estrogens (OR = 6.6; 95% CI, 3.1–12.6). The use of cyclical progestin reduced the risk dramatically (OR = 1.6; 95% CI, 1.1–2.4), but this risk increased in women who used the progestin for less than 16 days per cycle, most commonly 10 days per cycle (OR = 2.9; 95% CI, 1.8–4.6 for 5 or more years of use) (see Chapter 7)[49].

CONTROVERSIES IN ESTROGEN USE

HRT and 'hormonally dependent cancers'

The need for HRT in women with 'hormonally dependent cancers' is rather controversial. Since epidemiologic data showed the association of estrogen with an increase in the risk of developing breast and endometrial cancer, it has become an accepted dogma that estrogen administration, after the cancer has actually developed, may 'feed' that growth and compromise the patient's prognosis. Nonetheless, this assertion has not been substantiated by any published data associating estrogen with any detrimental effect on the course of cancer. This perceived dogma of avoidance of estrogen treatment in cancer survivors has been extrapolated from cell line growth kinetics and has enforced this clinical concept. It is interesting that these experimental data have not been considered in total, since estradiol for example may exhibit growth stimulatory effects at concentrations of 10^{-12} to 10^{-10} mol/l and inhibit the growth at 10^{-6} to 10^{-5} mol/l of a number of cancer cell lines[50].

HRT in survivors of breast cancer

For many years it was accepted that pregnancy endowed an adverse prognosis on breast cancer, an effect attributed to the high estrogen levels during pregnancy.

Indeed at some centers it was even regarded as an inoperable cancer owing to its rapid progress. This belief has now been dispelled, and survival of the breast cancer patient is similar – after correcting for age and stage – whether or not the patient is pregnant[51–53]. Furthermore, subsequent pregnancies do not increase the risk of recurrence, whether they occur within or beyond 2 years[52,54].

Ovariectomy used to be a major part of the treatment of breast cancer in premenopausal women, but it has failed the test of randomized clinical trials. Tamoxifen is an established adjuvant therapy in breast cancer and has been shown to reduce the rate of its recurrence. In premenopausal women it increases several-fold the endogenous production of estrogen during the menstrual cycle, yet tamoxifen is effective in reducing breast cancer recurrence. There seems to be no rationale for withholding estrogen replacement in these patients. An earlier report suggested an improved all-cause mortality in HRT users, including those who survived breast cancer. Furthermore, there are indications that survival of the breast cancer patient is better in those who use HRT[55]. A cohort study from Australia observed a death rate of 1.2% in HRT users compared to 11.5% in the whole database. When these data were corrected for confounding variables such as age, stage and parity the hazard ratio was 0.99 (95% CI, 0.40–2.47)[56], thus confirming earlier retrospective data[57–59] and case-controlled studies[60–62]. With the improved survival of breast cancer patients, the adverse effects of estrogen deficiency on quality of life and the risk of developing osteoporosis and cardiovascular disease have become more pressing issues, and many women demand more information. Current knowledge about the effect of estrogen on the prognosis of breast cancer must be shared with the patient, confirming that it is an option but stressing the fact that protection from recurrence can never be guaranteed.

Estrogen replacement following endometrial cancer

Removal of the ovaries during the surgical treatment of endometrial cancer removes a source of androgen, which is peripherally converted to estrone in postmenopausal women. This goes a long way to explaining the development of vasomotor symptoms in these patients postoperatively long after experiencing the menopause and the subsidence of these symptoms. The argument for withholding ERT from women who have undergone treatment for endometrial cancer is similar to that presented for breast cancer patients. This was initially challenged by Creasman and colleagues when they reported the recurrence of endometrial cancer in 2% of post-cancer estrogen users compared to 15% in the untreated group[63]. Even in those women with a high risk of recurrence (grade III and deep myometrial invasion) there were 26 deaths out of 174 non-estrogen users compared to one death out of 47 estrogen users after a minimum period of 5 years of follow-up. These data were subsequently confirmed by similar findings reported by other authors[64,65]. Despite the fact that all these studies were retrospective, it is generally felt that the use of postoperative estrogen in these patients, particularly those with stage I disease, is safe. The results of the ongoing double-blind study sponsored by the Gynaecology Oncology Group and the National Cancer Institute on the effectiveness and safety of ERT in patients who have suffered endometrial cancer will, it is hoped, establish a firm conclusion in this regard.

HRT and thromboembolism

Numerous publications have referred to the potential thrombogenic effect of ERT/HRT, and the argument surrounding these data is presented in Chapter 1. For premenopausal women who continue to menstruate following the thrombo-embolic incident, production of endogenous estrogen continues. The fact that, as index cases, they are more likely to develop another thromboembolic episode does not justify the surgical removal of their ovaries. Therefore, there is no rationale for not prescribing HRT in these women. It can be argued, however, that a non-oral route of administration may reduce the impact on liver synthesis of pro-coagulation factors. Nonetheless Goebelsmann and colleagues showed that it is the dose of estrogen rather than the route of administration that governs the rate of hepatic globin synthesis[7]. In addition a thromboembolic episode which follows trauma and prolonged immobilization is not likely to recur following hormone treatment. Moreover, those women on long-term warfarin treatment are already protected from recurrence, although warfarin induces the production of hepatic enzymes and may interfere with estrogen metabolism. Women should be counseled individually and encouraged to consider the advantages and disadvantages of commencing HRT.

The difficulty arises in those who develop deep vein thrombosis or a pulmonary embolus while taking HRT. These cases should be investigated thoroughly for factor V Leiden mutation and G20210A prothrombin mutations in addition to other pro-coagulation metabolic disorders and familial inheritance of protein S deficiency, for example (Table 9.2)[66].

The use of small doses of aspirin or low doses of warfarin has been advocated alongside a non-oral route of estrogen administration, but data are lacking regarding the effectiveness of this approach in protecting against recurrence. A significant number of women suffer so profoundly from their menopausal symptoms that

Table 9.2. Factor V Leiden mutation (activated protein C resistance), its prevalence and significance. Data from Bounameaux H. *Lancet* 2000;356:182–3[66]

	Isolated DVT	Isolated PE	DVT and PE	Controls
Prevalence (%)	15–18	4.9–12.1	13–24	2.8–5.3
Odds ratio (95% CI)	6.0 (4.6–7.8)	2.5 (1.8–3.5)	5.2 (3.6–7.5)	1.0

CI, confidence interval; DVT, deep vein thrombosis; PE, pulmonary embolism

they decide to go ahead with HRT, while others attempt to seek different remedies. Tibolone was reported not to change fibrinogen and plasminogen adversely, and although it is not licensed for this use and more data need to be generated in this regard, it may be a reasonable alternative.

CONCLUSIONS

The diagnosis of the menopause is easy but the contribution of estrogen deficiency to the total symptomatology of the perimenopausal woman may be difficult to evaluate. Commencing HRT in such patients can help to relieve these symptoms, but as many as 50% of them may experience menstrual irregularity and worsening of the symptoms of premenstrual tension.

The therapeutic options are based on the established effectiveness of estrogens, which have to be opposed by a progestogen in women with an intact uterus. A continuous combined estrogen/progestogen regimen may achieve amenorrhea in more than 50% of women, but its long-term cardiovascular safety is still to be documented.

The controversies surrounding the use of HRT in survivors of breast and endometrial cancer and those with a history of thromboembolism are discussed. Since the risk for developing any adverse event cannot be quantified in the individual woman, it is vital to educate women to enable them to make informed health choices.

REFERENCES

1. Prior JC. Perimenopause: the complex endocrinology of the menopausal transition. *Endocr Rev* 1998;19:397–428

2. Wallace RB, Sherman BM, Bean JA, *et al*. Probability of menopause with increasing duration of amenorrhea in middle-aged women. *Am J Obstet Gynecol* 1979;135:1021–4

3. MacNaughton J, Banah M, McCloud P, *et al*. Age related changes in follicle stimulating hormone, luteinizing hormone, oestradiol and immunoreactive inhibin in women of reproductive age. *Clin Endocrinol* 1992;36:339–45

4. Navot D, Rosenwaks Z, Margalioth EJ. Prognostic assessment of female fecundity. *Lancet* 1987;2:645–7

5. Winslow KL, Toner JP, Brzyski RG, *et al*. The gonadotropin-releasing hormone agonist stimulation test – a sensitive predictor of performance in the flare-up *in vitro* fertilization cycle. *Fertil Steril* 1991;56:711–17

6. Gulekli B, Bulbul Y, Onvural A, *et al*. Accuracy of ovarian reserve tests. *Hum Reprod* 1999;14:2822–6

7. Goebelsmann U, Mashchak CA, Mishell DR Jr. Comparison of hepatic impact of oral and vaginal administration of ethinyl estradiol. *Am J Obstet Gynecol* 1985;151:868–77

8. Mattsson LA, Christiansen C, Colau JC, *et al*. Clinical equivalence of intranasal and oral 17 beta-estradiol for postmenopausal symptoms. *Am J Obstet Gynecol* 2000;182:545–52

9. Sharp CA, Evans SF, Risteli L, *et al*. Effects of low- and conventional-dose transcutaneous HRT over 2 years on bone metabolism in younger and older postmenopausal women. *Eur J Clin Invest* 1996;26:763–71

10. Smith D, Prentice R, Thompson D, Herrman W. Association of exogenous estrogen and endometrial carcinoma. *N Engl J Med* 1975;293:1164–7

11. Hill GA, Wheeler JM. Incidence of breakthrough bleeding during oral contraceptive therapy. *J Reprod Med* 1991;36:334–9

12. Geusens P, Dequeker J, Gielen J, Schot LP. Non-linear increase in vertebral density induced by a synthetic steroid (Org OD 14) in women with established osteoporosis. *Maturitas* 1991;13:155–62

13. Bjarnason NH, Bjarnason K, Haarbo J, *et al*. Tibolone: prevention of bone loss in late postmenopausal women. *J Clin Endocrinol Metab* 1996;81:2419–22

14. Lippuner K, Haenggi W, Birkhaeuser MH, *et al*. Prevention of postmenopausal bone loss using tibolone or conventional peroral or transdermal hormone replacement therapy with 17 beta-estradiol and dydrogesterone. *J Bone Miner Res* 1997;12:806–12

15. Pavlov PW, Ginsburg J, Kicovic PM, *et al*. Double-blind, placebo-controlled study of the effects of tibolone on bone mineral density in postmenopausal osteoporotic women with and without previous fractures. *Gynecol Endocrinol* 1999;13:230–7

16. von Dadelszen P, Gillmer MD, Gray MD, *et al*. Endometrial hyperplasia and adenocarcinoma during tibolone (Livial) therapy. *Br J Obstet Gynaecol* 1994;101:158–61

17. Ramsay J, Calder A, Hart DM, *et al*. Hysteroscopic investigation of bleeding in women receiving tibolone: a case–control study. *Gynaecol Endosc* 1998;7:115–19

18. Habiba M, Ramsay J, Akkad A, *et al*. Immunohistochemical and hysteroscopic assessment of postmenopausal women with uterine bleeding whilst taking tibolone. *Eur J Obstet Gynecol Reprod Biol* 1996;66:45–9

19. Al-Azzawi F, Wahab M, Habiba M, *et al*. Continuous combined hormone replacement therapy compared with tibolone. *Obstet Gynecol* 1999;93:258–64

20. Bjarnason NH, Bjarnason K, Hassager C, Christiansen C. The response in spinal bone mass to tibolone treatment is related to bone turnover in elderly women. *Bone* 1997;20:151–5

21. Castelo-Branco C, Vicente JJ, Figueras F, *et al.* Comparative effects of estrogens plus androgens and tibolone on bone, lipid pattern and sexuality in postmenopausal women. *Maturitas* 2000;34:161–8

22. Delmas PD, Bjarnason NH, Mitlak BH, *et al.* Effects of raloxifene on bone mineral density, serum cholesterol concentrations, and uterine endometrium in post-menopausal women. *N Engl J Med* 1997;337:1641–7

23. Lufkin EG, Whitaker MD, Nickelsen T, *et al.* Treatment of established postmenopausal osteoporosis with raloxifene: a randomized trial. *J Bone Miner Res* 1998;13:1747–54

24. Walsh BW, Kuller LH, Wild RA, *et al.* Effects of raloxifene on serum lipids and coagulation factors in healthy postmenopausal women. *J Am Med Assoc* 1998; 279:1445–51

25. Ettinger B, Black DM, Mitlak BH, *et al.* Reduction of vertebral fracture risk in postmenopausal women with osteoporosis treated with raloxifene: results from a 3-year randomized clinical trial. *J Am Med Assoc* 1999;282:637–45

26. Wing RR, Matthews KA, Kuller LH, *et al.* Waist to hip ratio in middle-aged women. Associations with behavioral and psychosocial factors and with changes in cardiovascular risk factors. *Arterioscler Thromb* 1991;11:1250–7

27. Poehlman ET, Toth MJ, Fishman PS, *et al.* Sarcopenia in ageing humans: the impact of menopause and disease. *J Gerontol A Biol Sci Med Sci* 1995;50:73–7

28. Kushi LH, Folsom AR, Prineas RJ, *et al.* Dietary antioxidant vitamins and death from coronary heart disease in postmenopausal women. *N Engl J Med* 1996; 334:1156–62

29. Parazzini F, La Vecchia C, Bocciolone L, Franceschi S. The epidemiology of endometrial cancer. *Gynecol Oncol* 1991;41:1–16

30. Hunter D, Willett W. Re: dietary fat and breast cancer. *J Natl Cancer Inst* 1993;85:1776–7

31. Russo A, Franceschi S, La Vecchia C, *et al.* Body size and colorectal-cancer risk. *Int J Cancer* 1998;78:161–5

32. Franceschi S, Favero A, Decarli A, *et al.* Intake of macronutrients and risk of breast cancer. *Lancet* 1996;347:1351–6

33. Norman RJ, Flight IH, Rees MC. Oestrogen and progestogen hormone replacement therapy for peri-menopausal and post-menopausal women: weight and body fat distribution. *Cochrane Database Syst Rev* 2000;CD001018

34. Coleman MP, Babb P, Damiecki P, *et al. Cancer Survival Trends in England and Wales, 1971–1995: Deprivation and NHS Region.* London: Stationery Office Publications Centre, 1999

35. Colditz GA, Hankinson SE, Hunter DJ, *et al.* The use of estrogens and progestins, and the risk of breast cancer in postmenopausal women. *N Engl J Med* 1995;332: 1589–93

36. Ross RK, Paganini-Hill A, Gerkins VR, *et al.* A case–control study of menopausal estrogen therapy and breast cancer. *J Am Med Assoc* 1980;243:1635–9

37. McDonald JA, Weiss NS, Daling JR, *et al.* Menopausal estrogen use and the risk of breast cancer. *Breast Cancer Res Treat* 1986;7:193–9

38. Wingo PA, Layde PM, Lee NC, *et al.* The risk of breast cancer in postmenopausal women who have used estrogen replacement therapy [published erratum appears in *J Am Med Assoc* 1987;257:2438]. *J Am Med Assoc* 1987;257:209–15

39. Kaufman DW, Palmer JR, de Mouzon J, *et al.* Estrogen replacement therapy and the risk of breast cancer: results from the case-control surveillance study. *Am J Epidemiol* 1991; 134:1375–85; discussion 1396–401

40. Palmer JR, Rosenberg L, Clarke EA, *et al.* Breast cancer risk after estrogen replacement therapy: results from the Toronto Breast Cancer Study. *Am J Epidemiol* 1991;134: 1386–95

41. Sellers TA, Mink PJ, Cerhan JR, *et al.* The role of hormone replacement therapy in the risk for breast cancer and total mortality in women with a family history of breast cancer. *Ann Intern Med* 1997;127:973–80

42. Colditz GA, Egan KM, Stampfer MJ. Hormone replacement therapy and risk of breast cancer: results from epidemiologic studies. *Am J Obstet Gynecol* 1993;168: 1473–80

43. Danish National Board of Health. *Cancer Incidence in Denmark, 1996.* Copenhagen: Sunhedsstyrelsen, 1999

44. Collaborative Group on Hormonal Factors in Breast Cancer. Breast cancer and hormone replacement therapy: collaborative reanalysis of data from 51 epidemiological studies of 52,705 women with breast cancer and 108,411 women without breast cancer [published erratum appears in *Lancet* 1997;350:1484]. *Lancet* 1997;350:1047–59

45. Alexander FE, Anderson TJ, Brown HK, *et al.* 14 years of follow-up from the Edinburgh randomised trial of breast-cancer screening. *Lancet* 1999;353:1903–8

46. Kerlikowske K, Grady D, Rubin SM, *et al.* Efficacy of screening mammography. A meta-analysis. *J Am Med Assoc* 1995;273:149–54

47. Woodruff JD, Pickar JH. Incidence of endometrial hyperplasia in postmenopausal women taking conjugated estrogens (Premarin) with medroxyprogesterone acetate or conjugated estrogens alone. The Menopause Study Group. *Am J Obstet Gynecol* 1994;170:1213–23

48. Kurman RJ, Kaminski PF, Norris HJ. The behavior of endometrial hyperplasia. A long-term study of 'untreated' hyperplasia in 170 patients. *Cancer* 1985;56:403–12

49. Weiderpass E, Adami HO, Baron JA, *et al.* Risk of endometrial cancer following estrogen replacement with and without progestins. *J Natl Cancer Inst* 1999;91:1131–7

50. Fiorelli G, Picariello L, Martineti V, *et al.* Estrogen synthesis in human colon cancer epithelial cells. *J Steroid Biochem Mol Biol* 1999;71:223–30

51. Dow KH. Having children after breast cancer. *Cancer Pract* 1994;2:407–13

52. Dow KH, Harris JR, Roy C. Pregnancy after breast-conserving surgery and radiation therapy for breast cancer. *J Natl Cancer Inst Monogr* 1994;131–7

53. Higgins S, Haffty BG. Pregnancy and lactation after breast-conserving therapy for early stage breast cancer. *Cancer* 1994;73:2175–80

54. Zemlickis D, Lishner M, Degendorfer P, *et al.* Maternal and fetal outcome after breast cancer in pregnancy. *Am J Obstet Gynecol* 1992;166:781–7

55. Hunt K, Vessey M, McPherson K. Mortality in a cohort of long-term users of hormone replacement therapy: an updated analysis. *Br J Obstet Gynaecol* 1990;97:1080–6

56. Dew J, Eden JA, Beller E, *et al.* A cohort study of hormone replacement therapy given to women previously treated for breast cancer. *Climacteric* 1998;1:137–42

57. Stoll BA. Hormone replacement therapy for women with a past history of breast cancer. *Clin Oncol (R Coll Radiol)* 1990;2:309–12

58. Powles TJ, Hickish T, Casey S, O'Brien M. Hormone replacement after breast cancer. *Lancet* 1993;342:60–1

59. Vassilopoulou-Sellin R, Theriault T, Klein MJ. Estrogen replacement therapy in women with prior diagnosis and treatment for breast cancer. *Gynecol Oncol* 1997;65:89–93

60. Wile AG, Opfell RW, Margileth DA. Hormone replacement therapy in previously treated breast cancer patients. *Am J Surg* 1993;165:372–5

61. Eden JA, Bush T, Nand S, Wren BG. A case–control study of combined continuous estrogen–progestin replacement therapy among women with a personal history of breast cancer. *Menopause* 1995;2:67–72

62. DiSaia PJ, Grosen EA, Kurosaki T, *et al.* Hormone replacement therapy in breast cancer survivors: a cohort study. *Am J Obstet Gynecol* 1996;174:1494–8

63. Creasman WT, Henderson D, Hinshaw W, Clarke-Pearson DL. Estrogen replacement therapy in the patient treated for endometrial cancer. *Obstet Gynecol* 1986;67:326–30

64. Lee RB, Burke TW, Park RC. Estrogen replacement therapy following treatment for stage I endometrial carcinoma. *Gynecol Oncol* 1990;36:189–91

65. Chapman JA, DiSaia PH, Osann K, *et al.* Estrogen replacement in surgical stage I and II endometrial cancer survivors. *Am J Obstet Gynecol* 1996;175:1195–200

66. Bounameaux H. Factor V Leiden paradox: risk of deep vein thrombosis but not of pulmonary embolism. *Lancet* 2000;356:182–3

Index

interleukins, IL-1 and IL-6   8
Iowa Women's Health Study   154
ischemic heart disease   9

Leicester Endometrial Needle
    Sampler (LENS)   134–5
Leiden mutation, factor V   15, 158,
    159
levonorgestrel (LNG)   74
LNG-releasing vaginal device   148
    effects on endometrium   96–8
    long-term   96–7
    potency   80
lifestyle risk factors, endometrial
    cancer/neoplasia   115–16
linear discriminant analysis (LDA)
    99–103, 109
lipid monoclonal antibodies, estrogen
    effects   11–14
lipoproteins, estrogen deficiency
    11–14
luteal phase, endometrial histology
    93–5, 99–103
lynestrenol, structure   75

Macaca mulatta, model of
    progestogen–estrogen action   81
mammogenesis, in rat, optimal
    estrogen:progesterone ratio   77
mammography, screening   154
medroxyprogesterone acetate (MPA)
    and amenorrhea   22
    bleeding   25
    in Heart and Estrogen/Progestin
        Replacement Study (HERS)   15
    potency   78–80
    Pregnancy Maintenance test   78
menarche, early, risk factor for
    endometrial cancer/neoplasia   115

menopause
    diagnosis   145
    late, risk factor for endometrial
        cancer/neoplasia   115
    management   145–59
    pathophysiology   4–5
    treatment   146–52
    see also HRT
menstrual bleeding
    abnormal perimenopausal   107–9
    analysis   36–46
        definitions (WHO)   37
        graphical presentation   38–40
        numerical description   40–3
        regression modeling   43–6
    assessment methods   27–30
        regularity of intervals   29–30
    design of studies   35–6
    dysfunctional uterine bleeding
        (DUB)   108–9
    scheduled   23–5
    unscheduled (ccHRT)   25–7
menstruation   21–2
    and ethnicity   22
morphometry, endometrial   97–103
myocardial infarction   9

NADPH, pregnenolone production
    72
nestorone   75
norethindrone
    structure   75
    see also norethisterone (NET)
norethisterone (NET)   25
    conversion to ethinylestradiol   85
    efficacy   79–80
    potency   80
    Pregnancy Maintenance test   78
norethynodrel, structure   75